WHAT OTHERS AF
CONQUER YOUR PCOS NATURALLY

"Millions of women use medications on a daily basis to control their PCOS issues. When speaking with women they constantly tell me how sick and tired they are of being sick and tired. How they are fed up with the long list of side effects they experience from these medications. They want to go natural but don't know how. This book will help women understand how they can control their PCOS naturally. It is packed full of information to help you understand all aspects of the condition and how you can use alternative and/or natural therapies such as correcting vitamin/mineral deficiencies, beneficial foods/ways of eating, and a number of holistic treatments to control it and better your health. **This is a MUST read for anyone with PCOS,** whether they are trying to get pregnant or simply trying to control their condition."

> **– Pamela Pelletier, *PCOSInfo.com***

"My experience of PCOS is probably quite different to that of most women as I only started to have health issues after the birth of my second child. When my GP suspected I had PCOS she told me not to bother getting an "official" diagnosis as there was nothing that could be done to treat it, and just to get on with my life. Twelve months later after deciding I wanted to know for certain, the PCOS was confirmed, and the advice from my GP, knowing I didn't want any more children was the same as before, except I needed regular blood tests for diabetes and to exercise regularly because of my weight. The support from my GP was both inadequate and disappointing; this doctor was supposed to care and have the answers to help me achieve good health. I felt let-down. This lack of knowledge and understanding sent me in search for answers to help myself, and that is when Dr Rebecca Harwin and her incredible book *Conquer Your PCOS Naturally* came into my life. The information in this book is invaluable and has **provided me with the answers, insight and support that others could**

not. Being written by someone who had won the battle against PCOS has helped me to finally feel empowered to take control of my health, and provided me with the knowledge to do it. **This book is essential for anyone with PCOS,** and should be compulsory reading for every GP."

— **Jodie Barendsen,** *Ballarat, Australia*

"Conquer Your PCOS Naturally is an excellent book for anyone with this issue, and for those attempting to understand their partners and/or family members with this issue. As a woman with PCOS I can say from experience that once diagnosed, which could take many years, finding helpful, sound, information is difficult at best. One can certainly mine the internet for information, but be warned, you will be overwhelmed with an astounding amount of recommendations of supplements, medications, therapies and the like – none of which may work for your particular situation. While there are some books out there that address the issue of PCOS, almost all of them tend to give only basic, rudimentary education, and/or are focused on only one path to health. Some are only medically based, with information solely on diagnosis, causes, and medications, etc., while many more focus only on diet. While these are helpful, *Conquer Your PCOS Naturally* addresses PCOS, and your wellness, in its entirety. What does having PCOS mean? How does it affect your health, wellness, sense of self? Solid medical information about hormones, genes, and what medical tests you may want to take to find out more specifically about your unique situation with this disease is explained clearly and concisely. Dr Harwin continues on to look at your health and wellness as a whole, giving excellent advice on nutrition, stress management, food toxicity, supplements, exercise, and the holy grail for those of us trying to conceive, fertility. *Conquer Your PCOS Naturally* is **one of the best books I have read on the subject of PCOS** thus far and I highly recommend it to anyone that has this disease or wishes to learn more about it."

— **Dana Adams,** *New York City, USA*

"This book has been life-changing for me. I was diagnosed with PCOS in January of 2009 and have spent a lot of time online researching. The information found online is not always trustworthy or accurate. I felt so lost in a sea of information and, for over a year, felt too overwhelmed to actually do anything about my diagnosis. I figured there was medication out there for me whenever I decided to try and conceive and, other than that, I would just keep living like I was. Throughout reading this book, I have already begun to implement the food plans listed. I have noticed a change in both my mood and energy in just the past three weeks. I now understand what is happening to my body and what changes I need to make. The information is thoroughly researched and left me with no unanswered questions. **I feel now that I have the power to control my body,** instead of continuing to let my body control me. This book has given me the confidence to live my life in such a way that I will be able to reduce my risk of disease and improve my fertility. **Thank you, Dr Harwin, for such complete information on all things PCOS in this book!"**

– **Stacy Miller,** *Raleigh, USA*

"Dr Harwin has compiled a useful account of PCOS including her own journey which will serve as a guidebook for others suffering from this condition. Her holistic background offers a fresh perspective to the PCOS sufferer **giving hope** rather than just a mere label of disease. Dr Harwin reveals exciting news in the science of epigenetics emphasising that we are not victims of our genetics – rather we can control our health outcomes by our lifestyle decisions. **Reading this book is a must for anyone suffering from PCOS** as well as the health care provider looking to broaden their understanding of this condition!"

– **Dr Joel Fugleberg,** *Doctor of Chiropractic, Owner - Lifestyle Chiropractic*

About The Author

International author, PCOS expert and experienced clinician Dr Rebecca Harwin has been helping women improve their health for many years.

Dr Rebecca understands how tough it can be, having previously suffered with this syndrome herself. After overcoming each of the signs and symptoms and gaining the upper hand, she is excited to show you how to lose weight and keep it off, regain your period, boost your fertility, have healthier, clearer skin and conquer your PCOS.

Dr Rebecca has completed eight years of intensive University study, and holds three undergraduate degrees; a Bachelor of Chiropractic Science, a Bachelor of Applied Science (Clinical Science), and a Bachelor of Applied Science (Human Biology). She has also completed thousands of hours of further health studies.

She is passionate about combining her comprehensive education and research with her personal and clinical experiences to bring you a comprehensive way forward from PCOS to freedom.

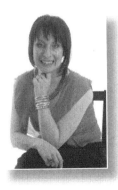

Conquer Your PCOS Naturally:
How to Balance Your Hormones, Naturally Regain Fertility and Live a Symptom-Free, Well Life

First published in Australia 2012 by The Publishing Queen
www.thepublishingqueen.com

ISBN 978-1-921673-61-0

Conquer *Your* PCOS

Poly | Cystic | Ovary | Syndrome

NATURALLY

How to Balance Your Hormones,
Naturally Regain Fertility and
Live a Symptom-Free, Well Life

DR REBECCA HARWIN
The PCOS Professional

Easy ways to follow Dr Rebecca!

You can get Dr Rebecca's PCOS related health tips, advice and thoughts by following her on:

Facebook at *Facebook.com/ConquerYourPCOS*
Become a fan and receive a special bonus:
'14 Daily Affirmations For Conquering Your PCOS'

Free downloads Don't forget to grab your special bonuses – FREE with the purchase of this book.

Visit **www.ConquerYourPCOSNaturally.com/BonusReports** to get your gifts – **worth $327!**

- *'Could The Medications You've Been Prescribed For Your PCOS Be Aggravating, Or Even Contributing, To Your Condition?'*
- *'What If The Foods Already In Your Cupboard Could Help You Conquer Your PCOS?'*
- *'Crush Male Infertility – How To Put The Lead In His Pencil And Improve The Quality Of His Lead'*
- **PLUS Receive The First THREE modules of 'Conquer Your PCOS' – The 12 Week Action Plan**

You'll also be automatically registered for your copy of Dr Rebecca's monthly newsletter *'Conquer Your PCOS'* – delivered straight to your inbox.

Keep up with the latest research, PCOS-friendly recipes, tips and insights, and special discounts and downloads available only to those who are a part of this inspired community.

Conquer *Your* PCOS
Poly Cystic Ovary Syndrome
NATURALLY

How to Balance Your Hormones,
Naturally Regain Fertility and
Live a Symptom-Free, Well Life

PLUS, Receive The First THREE Modules Of
'Conquer Your PCOS' – The 12 Week Action Plan

Dr Rebecca Harwin
The PCOS Professional

Dedication

To the beautiful women who suffer from PCOS.

You are my motivation and inspiration for writing this book.

This book has been written to educate, to encourage and to empower you to make the changes necessary to conquer your PCOS.

Acknowledgements

To my husband Dave, and Lincoln. Thank you for supporting me on my journey, and putting up with the long hours and occasional grumpiness that come with such a quest. For your hugs, laughs and saving my sanity! I love you both very much.

To my parents, Libby and Peter. For your support, your love and instilling in me the knowledge that one person can make a positive difference in our world. For your never-ending support and unwavering faith, thank you.

To my brother and sister, Ad and Rae. Blessed to have such incredible siblings whose support, belief, love and sense of humour mean the world to me.

To my extended family, Las, Mikaela and Chloe, Jacqui, Chris, Sue, Jo and Alfie. I feel so lucky to have you in my life and look forward to continuing on our journey together.

To Sam. A lifelong 'old' friend. I don't know if I have ever expressed how much I truly appreciate your friendship. Those exam baskets not only saved me from hunger and disaster, but let me know I was never alone.

To Dr Steven Hewitt. Your hugs, sense of humour, deep conversations and smile are priceless. Your skills as a Chiropractor and knowledge as a healer are inspirational.

To Rach. For your assistance and friendship. This book would not have been possible if it weren't for your help.

To Dr Kristie Lane. My peer mentor. Your guidance, challenging questions and friendship I truly appreciate. If you ever have the opportunity to be under her care, grab it with both hands.

To Dr Doug Herron. An inspiration. You have helped transform me into who I have become. I sincerely thank you.

To Kerry Watts. Personal Trainer extraordinaire. Thank you for your guidance, knowledge and friendship.

Last, but certainly not least, *to my patients and readers.* You are both my motivation and my inspiration, the force that kept me writing in those long, seemingly endless hours!

Contents

'I Was Scared I Would Have To Suffer From PCOS My Whole Life...'

I remember lying on the hospital table, embarrassed by bearing what I thought at the time was my fat belly. I was 17 years old and I had had excruciating tummy pain. The ultrasound gel felt cold, and I worried the pressure on my full belly might make me wet myself. The radiologist must have been doing rounds at the hospital, and he came in to take a look at my scans. He told me I had Poly Cystic Ovary Syndrome, but that was that. I didn't know what that meant, and it wasn't explained. I knew something wasn't 'normal', but I didn't know if I should even be worried, and he didn't seem overly concerned.

The next year I moved out of home to go to a University almost 2 hours away. The move from the country to the city, and away from my family, was really stressful. I often cried myself to sleep and I really missed home. I'm sure stress was a big factor in the further development of my PCOS. I put on almost 20kg and my self-esteem plummeted. I couldn't look in the mirror without cringing and feeling terrible about myself. My skin started to develop more spots and became more hairy. At least I saved what little money I had by not having to buy pads, after all, I had no period. I felt lost. No matter what I tried, I didn't seem to be able to lose weight or get my body back on track.

I went to see a gynaecologist praying for some answers. He was running 40 minutes late and I sat waiting awkwardly in his sterile office. After an impersonal 5 minute consultation, one I really couldn't afford as a student, he sat back on his chair, stared at me, and told me just to eat less and move more.

For many years, I suffered from hot flushes, dizzy spells, acne, excessive hair growth, weight gain and low self-esteem. I started to live in tracksuits as they were comfortable, and I thought they hid the fat. I couldn't find anyone with any expertise in PCOS. I just needed to know how to become healthy again, and I desperately wanted to no longer suffer from all of these symptoms.

My studies at University were science and health focused. Eight years in intensive university study gave me a great understanding of the human body and health. I also started to read other research, books and anything I could get my hands on, and I attended seminars often. I think my husband may describe me as a nerd. I worked out what PCOS really was, what it meant and what changes I needed to make to overcome it.

I vividly remember the first time I ovulated. For a second, I wondered what this sticky stuff in my knickers was. I was at the airport in Melbourne – sitting in the ladies with a smile so large I thought my face might crack! I was in my thirties. My skin has settled down, and I'm so grateful not to have a face full of spots. Getting my period is exciting and empowering. And I'm so happy I don't have those nauseating hot flushes or dizzy spells any more.

I knew many other women were suffering just as I had done and I also knew there was very limited accurate information available. I realised I had a responsibility to get this powerful information into the hands, minds and hearts of other women with PCOS.

This book is dedicated to helping you regain your health, boost your fertility, restore your period, lose excessive weight, and live a PCOS free life. I did it, and so can you.

Enjoy x

Dr Rebecca Harwin

Chapter One

What Is PCOS?

Plus, where to start

> *"The doctor of the future will give no medicine,*
> *but will interest his patients in the care of the human frame,*
> *in diet, and in the cause and prevention of disease."*
>
> Thomas Edison, Inventor

Introduction to Poly Cystic Ovary Syndrome (PCOS)

Firstly, I want you to know most of what you have been told about PCOS is probably wrong.

Secondly, I want you to understand the true meaning of 'health'. The World Health Organisation (WHO) definition states: "Health is not only the absence of infirmity and disease but also a state of physical, mental and social well-being." I must also add spiritual well-being. Symptoms may, or may not be a sign of disease. Lack of symptoms may, or may not be a sign of health. For example, if you have gastroenteritis and develop a fever, vomiting and diarrhoea, this is a completely healthy response by your body to kill and remove the invading bug. On the other hand, the first sign of heart dis-ease may be a fatal heart attack.

Addressing only one area of your life will not lead to the long-term glorious health you deserve in all areas of your life. Your body is an intricate web of complex interactions, based on simple truths and balance, and always innately intelligent responses. Throughout this book, you will see I refer to 'disease' as 'dis-ease' – not a horrible affliction, but a lack of ease in your body, mind and soul.

Your focus should be on what it takes to be optimally well. This is how you conquer your PCOS.

This book is *not* about which drugs work best. Looking at the cold hard facts, a lack of a pharmaceutical agent or agents is not the reason you are experiencing suboptimal health. The BEST medicine for PCOS, and the dis-eases you are more likely to experience as a result of it – heart dis-ease, cancer and diabetes – is positive lifestyle change. The research shows lifestyle improvements are superior to drug therapy, and far safer. These improvements focus on what it takes for a human being to be optimally well: movement, nutrition, thought and environment.

The history of PCOS

The first descriptions of PCOS date back to 1721. However, PCOS was first formally described in the mid-1930s by two Chicago doctors – Irving Stein and Michael Leventhal. The findings from their research were published in the *American Journal of Obstetrics and Gynaecology.* These doctors reported on women who were suffering from infertility, hirsutism (the excessive growth of thick dark hair in women), lacking a regular menstrual cycle, and with enlarged ovaries.

Stein and Leventhal developed a surgical intervention called a "wedge removal". This technique was successful in restoring ovulation. However, it did nothing to address the many other symptoms, or the underlying drivers, of PCOS.

As we have moved forward in time, treatments have revolved around the birth control pill, drugs to decrease 'male hormones' and, more recently, those that improve insulin sensitivity. However, these both bring about side effects and do not address the underlying drivers of dis-ease. It's a little like covering up your car's oil light, there to warn you there's a problem. Initially, it works – no more annoying light. But then, one day in the future, you wonder why your car no longer runs as it should. And what else has this low oil level done to your car's engine?

Increased emergence of PCOS

PCOS is present in up to 10% of Caucasian women and up to 15-20% of African-American and Hispanic women.

PCOS has been on the rise in recent years. This is attributable to our lifestyles. Excessive intakes of unhealthy food and drink, the introduction of artificial hormones to our food and environment, loss of appropriate nutrition, the constant state of stress we live under, suboptimal gut function, increasing medications, lack of movement and increasing rates of over-weight and obesity, are taking their toll on our physical, psychological and spiritual health.

Diagnosis

There are two main diagnostic criteria used for the diagnosis of PCOS; the Rotterdam Criteria and the NIH/NICHD. The Rotterdam criteria define PCOS as being present with at least two of the following: infrequent menstruation, excessive 'male' hormones (hyperandrogenism) and/or Poly Cystic ovaries on ultrasound. The NIH criteria define PCOS as the presence of hyperandrogenism and infrequent ovulation (oligo-ovulation). Both of these definitions are after the exclusion of other disorders that could be responsible for the symptomatic picture.

Pathophysiology of the ovary

Poly (meaning multiple) Cystic Ovary Syndrome (PCOS) got its name from the multiple 'cysts' in the ovaries. However, these 'cysts' are in actual fact immature follicles. Researchers (Hughesdon, Webber, Maciel) showed there is an increased number of growing follicles in a Poly Cystic Ovary (PCO). These egg follicles begin to develop, but may stop growing, known as 'follicular arrest'. If a dominant follicle does not enlarge and the egg does not mature, an egg is not released. This is known as anovulation, and affects hormonal balance. The numerous follicles also cause enlarged ovarian size.

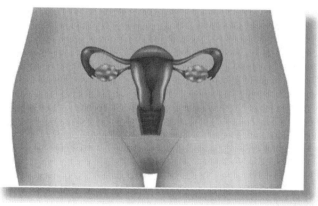

The appearance of Poly Cystic Ovaries
on either side of the uterus.

What does a Poly Cystic Ovary look like?

The definition of a Poly Cystic Ovary is one in which there is "either 12 or more follicles measuring 2-9mm in diameter and/or increased ovarian volume (>10cm^3)" [1]. The follicles appear in a typical peripheral pattern, also known as the 'string of pearls' appearance. This is most commonly determined by ultrasound – abdominal, and/or trans-vaginal. It's very important to have your scans performed by an experienced ultrasonographer. It is more accurate to have both abdominal and trans-vaginal scans performed. The trans-vaginal scan may not be performed if you are a virgin, or you refuse.

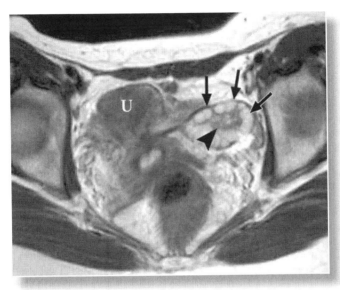

MRI image of multiple 'cysts', in a peripheral pattern, also known as the 'string of pearls' appearance.

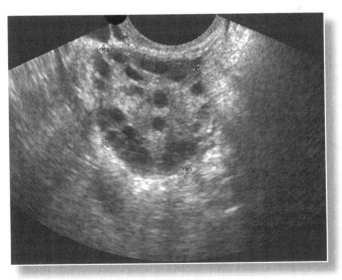

The appearance of a Poly Cystic Ovary under ultrasound.

What is the difference between Poly Cystic Ovaries and Poly Cystic Ovary Syndrome?

The appearance of Poly Cystic Ovaries, and Poly Cystic Ovary Syndrome, are two separate entities. A woman with the appearance of Poly Cystic Ovaries (PCO) may or may not have PCOS. Approximately 19-33% of the general female population[2] may show PCO appearance on an ultrasound.

Approximately 6-8% (although I have read many reports at up to 10%) of the female population has PCOS[3]. There is some thought that PCO may develop into PCOS given the 'right' conditions (i.e. weight gain, or an increase in insulin levels), however, until further research is conducted, these two entities should be considered distinct from one another. However, the lifestyle changes and advice in this book are not only what is best for a women with PCOS to be well, but also for a human being to be well. Regardless of whether you have PCO or PCOS, following the advice in this book will improve your health.

Symptoms

PCOS can present in a myriad of ways. The picture of an average woman with PCOS is of an overweight woman with irregular, potentially painful, periods, infertility, excessive facial and body hair and acne. However, there is much variation.

Symptoms may include:

- Delay of normal menstruation (primary amenorrhea)
- Fewer than normal periods (oligomenorrhea)
- Absent periods, after having previously experienced periods (secondary amenorrhea)
- Menstrual cycles without ovulation (anovulatory cycles)
- Painful periods with abnormal flow
- Excessive body and/or facial hair

- Male pattern balding (alopecia)
- Acne
- Poly Cystic Ovaries on ultrasound
- Infertility
- Overweight or obesity
- Difficulty losing weight
- Elevated insulin levels
- Skin discolouration (acanthosis nigricans)
- Skin tags
- Fatigue
- High blood pressure
- Abnormal blood lipid levels
- Cravings
- Mood swings
- Hot flushes
- Sleep apnoea
- Diabetes
- Heart dis-ease.

It's not just your ovaries

The name PCOS is somewhat misleading. It may lead you to believe this is an ovarian condition, but this is simply not the case. Your ovaries play an important role. However, PCOS is a 'whole body' endocrine condition, a systemic syndrome that affects the entire body.

Two of the main drivers of PCOS: Insulin Resistance and Inflammation

Insulin Resistance

One of the issues now known to lead to and aggravate PCOS

is Insulin Resistance. Your body produces insulin to allow your cells to 'take in' glucose. When a person's body cannot respond properly to the insulin, it produces excessive amounts – known as hyperinsulinemia. As hyperinsulinemia continues, Insulin Resistance results. The excess insulin causes the ovaries to swell and develop cysts, and stimulates secretion of excess amounts of androgen. These 'male hormones' affect regular ovulation, the menstrual cycle and cause the masculine characteristics associated with PCOS.

Implementing positive lifestyle changes will help you overcome Insulin Resistance. In this book, I will take you through the steps involved.

Inflammation

Inflammation is an underlying cause of dis-ease that is rarely discussed, let alone appropriately addressed. This is no different in women with PCOS, regardless of age[4]. Women with PCOS have been found to have elevated markers for inflammation[5]. Even before you begin to develop the tell-tale signs of PCOS, you may be suffering from chronic low grade inflammation affecting every part of your body.

The cure

"Why not adjust causes instead of treating effects?"

DD Palmer – Founder of modern day Chiropractic

The reality of the situation is this... you can take a variety of drugs to 'treat' each symptom, and then more to deal with the side effects. But, your body is not sick because of a lack of a drug. There is no miracle drug to cure PCOS. The only real way to overcome PCOS is lifestyle change. One truth remains constant for all human beings – what you eat, how you move, what you think and your environment, have dramatic effects on your body, mind and soul.

I congratulate you on taking the first incredibly important step – picking up this book. You must read this book from cover to cover, and then again. There is much to learn. There may be times when you think it's too complicated. If this happens, remember why you need to change. Remember also, everything comes down to a few simple points.

As a sufferer of PCOS, it is necessary to re-evaluate each aspect of your life. You need to create an environment conducive to a healthy life. The good news is the best lifestyle for a woman with PCOS is simply the same as the best lifestyle for any human being. You need to remove deficiency and toxicity and attain purity and sufficiency. By making healthy changes, you can conquer your PCOS, achieve a brand new state of optimal health, and create a happy, healthy, long life for yourself and your family.

Where to start?

If you are struggling to overcome your PCOS, are tired of being fobbed off and unable to find the answers to your deepest questions, you have picked up the right book at the right time. I will take you through – step by step – the information you need to know, including the steps you need to take, to conquer your PCOS.

This book has been written to educate, but especially to empower. I wish you all the very best of health, for now and into the future, for you, your family and the community we call our world.

Want access to your EXCLUSIVE downloadable bonuses?

Go to *www.ConquerYourPCOSNaturally.com/ BonusReports* now to get your 3 Bonus Reports:

'Could The Medications You've Been Prescribed For Your PCOS Be Aggravating, Or Even Contributing, To Your Condition?', 'What If The Foods Already In Your Cupboard Could Help You Conquer Your PCOS?' and *'Crush Male Infertility – How To Put The Lead In His Pencil And Improve The Quality Of His Lead'*

PLUS Receive The First THREE modules of 'Conquer Your PCOS' – The 12 Week Action Plan

Each part is complete and comprehensive. Loaded with in-depth information, regular contact and tips from myself, plus many other helpful bonuses. Learn how to change your life and *Conquer Your PCOS*, right from the comfort and privacy of your own home.

Absolutely FREE. Go now for instant access.

Chapter Two

Is PCOS In Your Genes?

*Learn how to control your genes
to be healthy instead of sick*

1.   Human genetics mumbo-jumbo!

We humans may be the 'magnum opus' of evolution. The process of evolution has endowed humans with unique capabilities that give us sovereignty over other species. However different we are in terms of nationalities, cultures and civilisations, we possess the same basic genetic framework. This is why we have similar body structures and similar physiological functions, despite the diversity of our appearance.

This has been so for thousands of years. It takes tens of thousands of years for a major genetic shift to occur in humans. Yet, humans are suffering ever increasing rates of 'disease' – heart dis-ease, cancer, diabetes and PCOS – at a rate much faster than our population growth. Let us consider only the past few hundred years... Given our genes haven't changed in that time, how is it possible to blame genes for the significantly increasing rates of dis-ease?

Less than 5% of dis-ease can be truthfully blamed on genetics. Yet, for many years, science and medicine have preached that our genetic material is the sole dictator of our lives, and 'disease', through a popular theory commonly known as 'the central dogma'. ARDictionary.com defines dogma as "a doctrinal notion asserted *without regard to evidence or the truth; an arbitrary dictum*". How true this is! This theory, thanks to the pioneering work of scientists like Dr Bruce Lipton, has been disproved. Sadly, this dangerous mistruth persists.

In this chapter, we will start our journey towards understanding the truth; the true role our genes play in our lives. You will learn what influences your genes. You will learn why environmental factors, which affect the development of PCOS in your life from 'womb' to 'grave', may affect future generations. We will also walk you through the genetic bare essentials.

All about genes

Before we discuss your genetic material in more depth, I want you to understand that each of the cells in your body has the same genetic information. Yet each tissue is structurally and functionally very different. In one location, we develop bone, in another muscle, in another brain, or breast or gut. The surrounding cells – and the environment they are in – determine which part of the genetic code is expressed, and which tissue they become. Although we have the same genetic material in each cell, a gene can be turned on or turned off, expressed or not. So, the next question begs – how can the expression of a gene be turned on or off? We'll come back to that soon.

All living beings, ranging from tiny viruses to giant elephants – carry a unique set of genes. Genes carry the blueprint for life – they code for the proteins necessary for us to respond and adapt to our constantly changing internal and external environment. Living beings of one species, be it a plant or an animal, share a similar genetic structure. Also, all organisms share some genes in common. The more common genes they have, the more they tend to resemble each other.[1] Ever wondered why chimpanzees and great apes are a lot like us?

In humans, genes are located in the compact central core called the 'nucleus' of every cell in our body. Genes are combinations of four chemicals called 'Nucleotide bases', which are arranged in long molecules called the DNA (Deoxyribo Nucleic Acid).

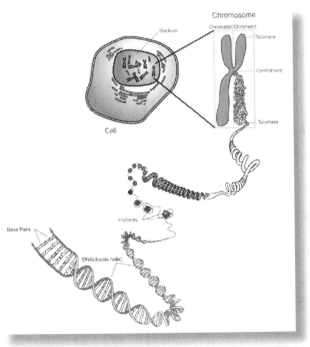

Structure of our chromosomes and DNA.

Picture from http://www.koshland-science-museum.org/exhibitdna/images/dna/

The four nucleotides are: A (adenine), C (cytosine), G (guanine) and T (thymine). The complex mixing and matching of these bases form DNA sequencing chunks. These chunks code for proteins, proteins that may give us a particular body feature or physiological function.

It is estimated humans have approximately 30,000 genes, or less. This is the same number as those in mice.[2] We and mice may share 99% similarity in our genes[3], yet we are so very different. That is because our genes become active at different times and under different circumstances. This changes development and response.

What is DNA?

DNA is arranged in two strands that lie parallel to each other, and contain the sequences of four nucleotide bases that form the genes. The structure of DNA actually looks like a spiral stair case. Every cell in our body carries the same DNA.

What are chromosomes?

Chromosomes are structures made of long strands of DNA and proteins. They are arranged in pairs and are carried in the nucleus of our cells. Humans have 46 chromosomes arranged in 23 pairs. A large number of genes are carried on each chromosome. The aggregate of genes carried on all of the 23 pairs makes for our genome. About 3% of this genome actually contains genes. These regions are called 'coding regions',

As compared to 23 pairs of chromosomes in humans, a donkey has 31, a hedgehog has 44, and a fruit fly has just 4 pairs of chromosomes!

http://www.medicalnewstoday.com/articles/120574.php

and they are scattered throughout the chromosomes. About 97% of the genome contains non-coding regions, (i.e. regions that are not genes). The functions of these non-coding regions were initially ignored, labelled 'junk DNA'.[4] However, advanced research has proven that these non-coding regions perform important functions affecting the function of our genes.

Where do our genes come from?

We inherit our genetic material from our parents. Each of our cells carry 23 pairs of gene bearing chromosomes; a total of 46 chromosomes. During the process of fertilisation, sperm from the father carrying 23 chromosomes met the egg from the mother carrying 23 chromosomes. When the sperm fertilises the ovum, their genetic material fuses to form a complete set of 46 chromosomes.

Thus, we get half of our chromosomes from our father and half from our mother.[5]

How do we pass on our genes?

When we conceive a child, we pass on our genetic material to them. Men pass their genes via their sperm and women do so via their ova or eggs. These tiny cells combine to form a baby. Even after we die, we still continue to 'survive' for many generations through our genes.[6]

How do genes work?

An individual's genetic make-up is called their 'genotype'. The characteristics that the genes code for (e.g. eye colour, or hair curl) are called their 'phenotype'. Each gene provides the code for a particular protein, which allows the performance of a specific function.

Some genes code for structural characteristics that enable cells to differentiate into muscle, skin or bone in one place, and heart, brain or gut in another. Other genes help us sustain life by coding for hormones like insulin, or important blood factors like haemoglobin.[7]

We carry thousands of genes but not all of our genes are 'switched on' at the same time. Genes are 'turned on' and 'turned off', as and when a particular protein is needed. The structures in our DNA, which determine the expression of genes, are called 'regulatory sequences'. These sequences do not code for the production of proteins. They regulate the expression – that is the 'turning on' and 'turning off' – of genes. These sequences are like 'switches' that determine whether the code on a gene will be made available to the cell's gene transcription apparatus or not[8] – whether the genetic page will be available to the reader.

Now, the important part – genes by themselves are just a set of instructions. For a gene to produce the protein it is coded for, it needs an order. These orders come from various sources, mostly – our lifestyle and the environment that we live in.

Think about wound healing. We have genes that are triggered to produce the substances needed for healing. However, they are 'turned on' only when we are injured. They are 'turned off' once the injury has healed, as that function is no longer needed. This is innate intelligence! Environmental factors are responsible for your genetic expression. As Dawson Church has beautifully quoted in his book *The Genie in Your Genes* – "In reality, genes contribute to our characteristics, but do not determine them."[9]

2.   The central dogma hoax

The claim that genes alone determine our fate is nothing more than fallacy. There are many factors – diet, how we move, how we think, how much we sleep, other lifestyle choices and our environment – that are pivotal in determining which genes are expressed or hidden, and when. These factors radically change our growth, our development and our health.

Let's have a closer look.

For years, we have been told authoritatively by 'experts' that our genes are the *brains* of the cell, that they control the cell, and so control our health.

If this was the case, removing the genes – the cell brain – from a cell, should cause instantaneous death to the cell, yes?

Dr Bruce Lipton, a PhD cellular biologist, is an expert in this area. He conducted experiments, removing the nucleus (the home of the genes) from a cell. The cell lived on.

In other research, he took genetically identical cells and placed them in three different environments. Amazingly, they produced different tissue.[10] The environment the cells were in determined the tissue they became – not the genes. He has shown the environment, working through the cell membrane (the walls of the house, so to speak), turn the genes – our genes – on or off. This has amazing, and exciting repercussions. After all, if our genes are in control, and we can't control our genes, we can't control our health... We would need drugs, surgery, someone outside of ourselves, to control these destructive genes for us, to prevent our demise from inevitable genetically predetermined disease.

> *"In a diverse array of popular sources, the gene has become a supergene, an almost supernatural entity that has the power to define identity, determine human affairs, dictate human relationships, and explain social problems. In this construct, human beings in all their complexity are seen as a product of a molecular text... the secular equivalent of a soul – the immortal site of true self and determiner of fate."*
>
> The DNA Mystique,
> by Dorothy Nelkin

However, Dr Lipton and others have proven the current 'genetic' theory of control (known as 'the central dogma') to be incorrect.

If you are a pharmaceutical company, this is bad news. After all, if all diseases are genetic, there is no other option than drugs and surgery. For sufferers of PCOS (and other dis-ease), Bruce Lipton's work is *wonderful news*. After all, if the genes do not control the cell, there must be something else. The exciting part is that this *something else* is under *our* control.

Just like the cells in Dr Lipton's experiment, our genes and cells respond to the environment we provide them. If we have a healthy lifestyle, we promote healthy gene expression and therefore well-being. If our lifestyle is not that which we are designed for, we promote adaptive gene expression – our body continues to try to adapt to the suboptimal environment we are providing it, leading to fatigue and eventually death...

What does this mean for you?

Nurture is far more important than nature. In fact, nurture causes nature. You are in control of your health.

Many clinicians cling to the antiquated belief that your genes determine your health. Given our genetic makeup has not changed markedly in the past 40,000 years, how is it then that the incidence of dis-ease has increased steeply in the past hundred years? What has changed if not our genes? The answer to this question is that our living conditions and lifestyle has changed drastically during this period. It is the changed environmental conditions that are causing dis-ease. What we need to look at is what affects the expression of our genes? This is the field of Epigenetics.

'Epigenetics' means 'above genetics'. It is the study of what causes a gene to be turned on, or turned off. These changes do not change the structure of the genes; but they significantly change the way these genes are expressed, or not. Epigenetic factors like lifestyle, diet, environmental factors like the air we breathe, water we drink, stress, smoking and so on can affect the way our genes behave for the better or for the worse.[11]

Changes in the gene expression due to epigenetic factors are reversible and sometimes stable. Importantly, these changes are heritable i.e. they can be passed from parents to children.[12] The developmental biologist Conrad Hal Waddington first defined the term 'Epigenetics' in 1942. His research helped to shift our focus from 'gene worship' back to the changes in our lifestyles and our environment that were directly influencing our genetic expression.

> *"As bizarre as it might sound, what you eat or smoke today could affect the health and behaviour of your great grand children."*
>
> Ethan Walters,
> Discover *magazine*

Scientists who have studied Epigenetics have found that we have two types of information – genetic and epigenetic. The genetic material influences the protein production, while the epigenetic information provides instructions on how, where and when the genetic information should be deployed.[13] Remember, the genes are simply the recipe. The chef and the ingredients matter, and determine the success of the recipe.

How do epigenetic factors work?

Two important mechanisms by which epigenetics affect our genetic expression are DNA methylation and histone modification.

Our DNA can be 'decorated' with chemical labels that affect the expression of genes without changing the structure of the DNA.[14] Chemicals like the methyl groups and histones come into play due to various epigenetic factors:

DNA methylation: The methyl groups present in a cell can be attached or removed from a certain area of the DNA, depending on the environment presented to the cells. This methyl group can act to switch on, or switch off, the expression of a gene. They can essentially open the genetic page to be read (switched on), or keep the page closed so it cannot be read (switched off). High levels of methyl groups in the gene regulatory regions of the DNA can lead to lowered transcription of certain genes.[15] Due to their tremendous influence over the functions of genes, methyl groups are included under epigenetic factors. Abnormal methylation of genes often occurs during the transformation of normal cells to cancer cells and is often found in cervical, prostate, colon, thyroid, stomach and breast cancers.[16]

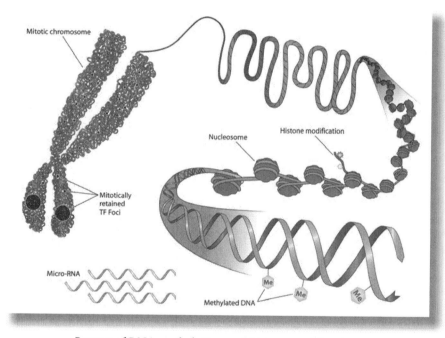

Process of DNA methylation and histone modification.

Picture from http://mcb.asm.org/content/30/20/4758/F1.expansion.html

Histone modification: Histones are a kind of protein present in our cell nuclei. They act as spools around which the DNA winds and coils itself to form compact structures. Histones help to make our DNA compact enough to fit into the tiny cell nucleus. Epigenetic factors bring about chemical changes in the cell nucleus. These chemicals bind to the histones on specific sites and change the availability of certain genes in our DNA for transcription. By doing so, they regulate the 'turning on' and 'turning off' of these genes.

Why should you be aware of epigenetics?

Women suffering from PCOS are often told that PCOS is genetic, that they are destined to suffer. However, we know otherwise. By understanding the factors that can promote optimal gene expression, and knowing the effect that your lifestyle choices exert – both beneficial and otherwise – you can give your life a complete makeover. With knowledge, you can make positive changes in your lifestyle. This will affect the genes you express and positively affect your health.

"In the past, diseases like cancer and heart disease were 'known' to be caused by the bad genes people inherited from their parents. However, the fact is that only 5% of patients could attribute their disease to heredity."

Willett WC, 2002

Studies like those performed by Dr Lipton are not simply a ray of hope, but warm sunshine bursting through, at times, desolate clouds. To all women with PCOS, who have given up hope, thinking that PCOS is the fault of your genes... you can turn your life around! By taking positive steps to live as nature intended, you can begin the transformation from victim to healthy warrior, conquering not just your symptoms and pain, but preventing PCOS from affecting your life, and the lives of your future generations.

3.   Epigenetic spin on PCOS

PCOS is a very complex metabolic syndrome and the extent to which we understand it may be just the tip of the iceberg. During the past decade, more than 100 genes have been studied for their association with PCOS, yet no single gene or group of genes have been universally accepted as major contributors to PCOS.

Researchers have come to accept that PCOS materialises and progresses due to a complex interplay between genetic and epigenetic factors.[17]

I had an opportunity to attend 'The 2nd Nutritional Genomics Symposium: A Healthy Start to Life'. Cutting edge research was presented on how nutrients/diet affects our genetic expression. One of the studies looked at how certain genes (including some that code for insulin signalling) are expressed in the babies of mothers who are overweight or dieting around the time of conception. The researchers found that liver insulin sensitivity was decreased in babies of overweight mothers. Wow! Shocking as it is, being overweight, or dieting around conception, actually changes the expression of insulin signalling genes in the babies in utero.[18] As you will learn throughout this book, insulin sensitivity is very important in women with PCOS.

This piece of information is precious to women looking to have children. It means that their PCOS can influence the expression of their baby's genes right from the womb. Their baby's future life may be affected from the time they are conceived. If you consider a female baby is developing her eggs while she is in the mother's womb, you can see the importance of your behaviours on future generations. This information is not meant to shock, but educate. Making the appropriate lifestyle changes prior to conception is a potent step toward health – for both the mother and her future baby.

Research studies have consistently shown that a mother's diet before conception, around the period of conception, during pregnancy and during breastfeeding has profound effects on the expression of genes in their babies. These epigenetic factors can increase or decrease the risk of dis-eases like obesity, cancer, heart dis-ease, PCOS and type-2 diabetes in the children.[19]

Dana Dolinoy's work with agouti mice provides further evidence for the importance of nutrition and a healthy baby. These mice got the rough end of the genetic stick, so to speak. They developed obesity, suffered from heart dis-ease and stroke, and died young. This 'bad stroke of luck' could be linked to a specific bunch of genes. However, even though these poor mice got a bad bunch of genes, there was more to the story... When the environment in the pregnant mother's womb was changed, the genetic expression in the baby mouse was changed. When the mother received methyl group rich supplements, such as folic acid and vitamin B12, the baby mice no longer developed obesity, and stopped dying early from the dis-eases they seemed genetically predetermined to die from.[20]

Now remember, the inherited genes did not change – the expression of the genes did. And it was nutrition and the environment that caused the change.

In women suffering from PCOS, central obesity and a dominance of 'male' hormones, an environment is created that favours PCOS during conception and in the early development of the baby in their uterus. Maternal androgen excess can even make the ovarian cells in the baby differentiate into cells that are similar to those in male testis (Leydig cells), further contributing to the PCOS development.[21] These epigenetic factors can also influence the distribution of fat in the body of the foetus and make the baby prone to central obesity later in life.[22]

Why should you be aware of this scientific mumbo-jumbo?

A little knowledge goes a long way. Early changes in lifestyle and diet will help you tackle, or even pre-empt, obesity and Insulin Resistance. These changes can aid in the prevention of PCOS complications like type 2 diabetes, cardiovascular dis-ease and cancer. In women with PCOS, lifestyle and food modifications will help to overcome the symptoms of PCOS. More importantly, these changes will lead to true health, well-being and vitality. The advice given in this book nourishes your best genetic expression.

Remember: Your body is a remarkable powerhouse. *Your body is self-healing, self-regulating and innately knowledgeable.* Having the blessed position of being a Chiropractor, I have long known and respected the power that made the body, heals the body. You simply need all the necessary building blocks – and no interference – to produce the glowing health you deserve. Your genes are not in control, you are. Epigenetics simply confirms this.

As Dawson Church says in his book *The Genie in Your Genes*[23] – "The tools of our consciousness – including our beliefs, prayers, thoughts, intentions and faith – often correlate much more strongly with our health, longevity and happiness than our genes do!"

Can't get enough?

Go to *www.ConquerYourPCOSNaturally.com/ BonusReports* to grab your FREE bonuses.

As an additional bonus, you'll also receive Dr Rebecca's *'Conquer Your PCOS'* monthly newsletter for FREE. You'll discover even more PCOS advice, easy-to-apply practical tips, PCOS-friendly recipes, and become a *'Conquer Your PCOS'* VIP.

Act now and join us and the 'Conquer Your PCOS' community!

Chapter Three

Restore Your Hormonal Balance

Discover what your hormones do, how they affect your PCOS, and the secrets to balancing them once more.

Your Hormones

One of my patients with PCOS had her ovaries removed after being diagnosed with ovarian cancer. She asked me, "So now that my ovaries have gone, does that mean my PCOS has gone too?" My answer was 'no'. Removing her ovaries might have 'cured' her of the ovarian cysts, but it did not entirely cure the underlying culprit. Poly Cystic Ovaries are only one aspect of PCOS.

> *"If hormones are making their presence known in your life, it is best to give them the attention they want."*
>
> *Geoffrey Redmond,*
> It's Your Hormones.

Our body is such a complicated web of chemical communications, and the functions of our hormones are closely intertwined with one another. PCOS has a medley of out-of-sync hormones, ranging from well-known hormones like insulin, testosterone and oestrogen, to lesser known hormones such as Luteinising Hormone (LH) and Follicle Stimulating Hormone

(FSH). If you are to conquer your PCOS, you need to know what your hormones are doing and how YOU can balance their functions.

What are hormones?

Hormones are chemical messengers used by the trillions of cells we each have in our body. Hormones are one of the languages our cells use to communicate with each other, in order to work in an organised and unified manner. They have tremendous control over the functioning of every system in our body and also our mind. Hormones are unique in that they exert their actions on organs that are far away from where they are produced.

Where do hormones come from?

Hormones are secreted by specialised glands in our body known as 'endocrine glands'. These glands include the hypothalamus, pituitary, pineal, thyroid, parathyroid, adrenals, pancreas (Islets of Langerhans), and the gonads, which are the testes in men and ovaries in women. With any changes in our inner or outer environment, these glands release hormones that travel through our bloodstream, telling our cells how to respond.[1]

How do hormones work?

Hormones have specific shapes that can fit into a specialised area on and in our cells, called a 'receptor'. These hormones fit into areas like a key in a lock and trigger, or stop, specific functions. Every cell has many different receptors, each reserved for a specific hormone.

Hormones interact with each other in a complex manner. The levels of our hormones are relative to each other. They maintain their levels by using what are called 'feedback loops'. In simple words, each hormone has a signalling system to communicate with other hormones, and their glands. They can control the levels of other hormones by facilitating the secretion of some, while stopping the function of others. Your body is innately working to maintain a dynamic balance – called 'homeostasis' – of your hormones. It is always trying to keep you safe. However, when chronic hormonal imbalances occur in response to an imbalanced lifestyle, syndromes like PCOS can materialise.

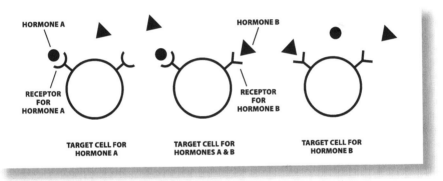

Hormones and receptors.
Original image provided with permission by www.FTMguide.org

Why learn about hormones?

Hormonal balance is essential for your well-being, growth, development, metabolism, brain function, sexual and reproductive functions and much more. To cut a long story short – your hormones are very important. Learning about your hormones will give you an understanding of what's happening to your body, and will give you the much needed confidence to change your health for the better. Good professional guidance can be critical, but there is no substitute for being the master of your own health – for taking the health reins in your own hands.

When suffering from a complicated hormonal disorder like PCOS, it is important that you understand how your body functions, the effect your hormones have and the steps that you can take to reclaim your hormonal balance. The following section will equip you with the knowledge you need in your crusade against PCOS.

Your hormones and PCOS

The hormonal imbalance of PCOS may present as vague signs and symptoms. Even experienced health practitioners can misdiagnose PCOS due to its many presentations. You may have mild symptoms, or severe. Vague symptoms, or definite. In this section we will discuss the hormones – and other important factors – involved in the development of PCOS, and the steps you need to take to restore your hormonal balance.

The hormonal culprits of PCOS

Insulin

Insulin is a very important hormone secreted by the pancreas in our abdomen. Insulin controls the processing of carbohydrates and proteins and is responsible for metabolism and storage of fat.[2] All our body cells require

Eleven signs of hormonal imbalance in women:

- *PMS and changes in menstruation*
- *Acne, oily skin and excessive hair growth*
- *Dizziness*
- *Fatigue*
- *Low sex drive*
- *Anxiety and depression*
- *Weight gain*
- *Urinary tract infections (UTIs)*
- *Headaches*
- *Allergies*
- *PCOS*

glucose for energy production, and insulin is the hormone that helps it move from our blood and into our cells.

Insulin Resistance (IR): Insulin Resistance is a condition where our cells can neither correctly recognise nor use the hormone insulin. Some women are more prone to Insulin Resistance (Asian and black women), however, faulty diet, lifestyle and excessive stress can cause it. Insulin Resistance is a major driver in PCOS. Between 44 to 70% of women with PCOS suffer from Insulin Resistance, irrespective of whether they are overweight or slender.[3] However, women who are obese have an increased risk of developing Insulin Resistance.[4]

You are most likely to develop Insulin Resistance if you are:

- *Overweight, with a Body Mass Index (BMI) more than 25*
- *40 plus years of age*
- *Have a waistline more than 35 inches/88cm**
- *Have PCOS*
- *Have high blood pressure and/or heart dis-ease*

* Use of Waist Circumference to Predict Insulin Resistance: Retrospective Study, by *Wahrenberg H, Hertel K, et al. BMJ. 2005; 11: 330:1363-1364.*

A diet laden with sugars, empty calories, unhealthy fats and processed foods, combined with stress and a lack of movement lowers our body's sensitivity to normal levels of insulin over a period of time. Our cells have special sites in which the molecules of insulin fit like the pieces of a jigsaw puzzle. In Insulin Resistance, there is a malfunctioning of these sites, so they cannot bind optimally with insulin. They stop responding to normal insulin levels and cannot remove glucose from our blood as they should. High blood sugar levels force our pancreas to produce more insulin, in an attempt to manage the increasing blood sugar. This leads to a condition where there is too much insulin in our blood, called 'hyperinsulinemia'.[5]

How does Insulin Resistance/hyperinsulinemia cause PCOS?

Insulin Resistance has a two-fold effect in PCOS. On one hand, Insulin Resistance increases the secretion of testosterone from the ovaries. On the other hand, it reduces the production of Sex Hormone Binding Globulin (SHBG), which is required for neutralising excessive testosterone in our blood.[6] Excessive free testosterone in the blood can further increase Insulin Resistance[7], creating a vicious cycle.

Due to its dual effect, Insulin Resistance can both cause, as well as amplify, the symptoms of PCOS. It is a major culprit behind the central obesity in women with PCOS. Additionally, Insulin Resistance can prevent the ovaries from producing ova or eggs, leading to anovulation and infertility.[8]

Finally, there is a theory that insulin directly causes excessive adrenal androgen production and favours the hypo-pituitary-gonadal axis (HPG-axis) disorder in PCOS, and is thereby directly responsible for aggravating PCOS.

Tell-tale signs of Insulin Resistance

- Central obesity
- Skin tags
- Abnormal skin pigmentation – *acanthosis nigricans*
- Acne
- Excessive hair on face and body (and/or loss of hair from the scalp)
- Irregular or absent periods

- Increased triglycerides and/or high blood pressure
- Intestinal bloating
- Sugar cravings
- Fatigue and/or brain fogginess and/or depression and/or mood swings.

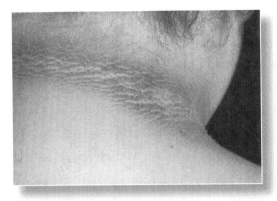

Acanthosis nigricans.
Source: dermatology.cdlib.org

Diagnosis of Insulin Resistance

Diagnosis may include tests like the two-hour glucose tolerance test, fasting blood glucose and insulin testing.[9]

Dangers of Insulin Resistance

If Insulin Resistance is not managed in its early stages, you can be at a greater risk of developing heart dis-ease, metabolic syndrome, type-2 diabetes, sleep apnoea, fatty liver dis-ease and endometrial cancer.[10,11]

Tackling Insulin Resistance

Lifestyle improvement is your most powerful weapon against Insulin Resistance. A well-balanced food plan and physical activity are effective ways of improving your insulin sensitivity. I discuss how to improve your lifestyle throughout this book. As an added perk, these lifestyle modifications will also improve your fertility.[12] Ensuring enough sleep, managing your stress levels, maintaining healthy levels of physical activity, the food plan recommended throughout this book and supplementation with nutrients such as fish oil, chromium and magnesium are vital in overcoming Insulin Resistance.

Testosterone

Testosterone is thought of as a 'male hormone' as men produce 10 times more testosterone than women. Male hormones are collectively called 'androgens'. We women need a little bit of male hormone too. Testosterone is needed for normal sexual function in both men and women.[13] In women, this hormone is normally produced by the ovaries and adrenal glands.

Too much testosterone = PCOS?

For many women, an excessive blood testosterone level – total and/or free testosterone (hyperandrogenism) – is one of the hallmarks of their PCOS, and part of the diagnostic criteria.

The excess testosterone in PCOS is due to two mechanisms. Abnormally high levels of the hormone LH (secreted by the pituitary) causes an imbalance in the hypothalamus-pituitary-ovarian axis (the way your brain talks to your ovaries). High LH levels coax the ovaries to produce more testosterone by developing cysts and causing thickening in ovarian tissues.[14] The second mechanism is Insulin Resistance, which triggers abnormal testosterone production. It also prevents its removal from the blood by reducing the testosterone binding globulin - Sex Hormone Binding Globulin (SHBG), thus leaving too much free male hormone in the body.[15] Excess body weight and obesity can also contribute to excessive testosterone production. Fat tissue contains enzymes that can produce testosterone (from its chemical precursors).[16]

Too much testosterone not only contributes to PCOS, but it can also lead to various psychological disturbances such as depression and mood disorders.[17]

Tell-tale signs of testosterone excess

- Hirsutism – thick hair growth on the chin, upper lip, chest, abdomen and back
- Acne
- Male pattern balding of the scalp hair
- Deepening of the voice
- Abnormal or absent menses
- Mood disturbances and depression.

Ways of calming down raging testosterone

Conventional treatments with synthetic medicines may help reduce testosterone levels. However, you must understand that these easy options come at the cost of your health and do not address the underlying drivers of PCOS.

The best and safest way to balance testosterone levels is to adopt a healthy lifestyle. Improving your insulin sensitivity and reducing excess body weight, if needed, combined with a healthy food plan and suitable physical activity will slowly yet surely rid your body of excess testosterone.

Typical western foods rich in unhealthy fats and carbo-hydrates favour testosterone production. Research shows dietary changes play a major role in balancing the levels of hormones in women. A study conducted in Milan, Italy showed substituting meats, eggs and dairy products with vegetarian sources of nutrients like fruits, vegetables, whole grains and legumes, significantly reduced the levels of excess testosterone in women. Refined carbohydrates like sugar, white bread and refined flour should be avoided. Consuming at least one portion of organic soy products like tofu, miso, or tempeh can provide you with natural plant hormones or phytoestrogens, which may help in balancing your hormones. Fish cooked with minimal oil or fat, seaweed, and flaxseeds (linseeds) are some other foods found to be helpful. These food changes also increase the levels of SHBG, which is required to inactivate excess active testosterone.[18]

Decrease or eliminate your alcohol consumption. Alcohol has also been shown to increase the levels of plasma dehydroepiandrosterone sulfate – a weak male hormone in women.[19]

Liquorice root *(glycyrrhiza)* has also been shown to be effective in decreasing testosterone levels. Research by P. Bergner in *Medical Herbalism* showed a significant reduction of circulating testosterone in women with PCOS with liquorice root.

What tests can be done?

Total testosterone and free/bio-available testosterone are two blood tests taken to check testosterone levels. Tests to detect SHBG levels should also be performed.[20]

Sex Hormone Binding Globulin (SHBG)

SHBG is a glycoprotein that serves as an escort for testosterone, oestrogen and progesterone, once they are in the blood. It functions to bind excessive circulating steroid hormones, and inactivate them, thereby maintaining their concentration in our blood.[21] SHBG shows more affinity in binding with androgens than oestrogens. SHBG is produced mainly by our liver and in some amounts by the breast tissue in women.[22] Oestrogen stimulates, while testosterone inhibits the production of SHBG.

Women naturally have higher levels of SHBG as compared to men, which help to keep testosterone levels in women in balance.[23]

The SHBG and PCOS connection

Women with PCOS often have low levels of SHBG. This increases the levels of free, or active, testosterone in the blood.

Insulin Resistance and high levels of insulin (hyperinsulinemia) are believed to lead to a lowered SHBG production in PCOS. Women with diabetes also suffer from Insulin Resistance, which leads to lowered SHBG levels.[24] In fact, studies have shown that low SHBG levels can be considered an integrated marker for Insulin Resistance. Increased testosterone production by the ovaries, adrenals and fatty tissue in obese women with PCOS may also contribute. More fat, especially around the belly, can lower your SHBG levels.[25] Women with lowered thyroid hormones (i.e. hypothyroidism) also have low SHBG levels.

Tell-tale signs of low SHBG

Look for the same signs as those seen in increased testosterone levels i.e. hirsutism, acne, a disturbed menstrual cycle etc.

What tests need to be taken?

Blood tests to detect the SHBG levels should be performed along with tests to detect total and free testosterone in women with PCOS. These tests collectively give a clear picture of your SHBG levels, and their impact on your testosterone levels.

How to boost SHBG levels naturally

An appropriate food plan and physical activity improves insulin sensitivity, reduces excess testosterone and helps you lose weight. It will also give you the additional benefit of boosting your SHBG levels. You should know that SHBG and body weight are inversely related to each other, meaning the higher your body weight, the lower your SHBG level will be.

Vegetarian food plans rank high when it comes to improving the hormonal balance in PCOS. Women who eat a lot of high fibre vegetables and fruits have higher levels of SHBG. Also, diets low in meats and dairy may promote higher SHBG levels.[26]

Oestrogen

Oestrogen is produced mainly by the ovaries, and also by the placenta during pregnancy.

It is vital for the development of the breasts, widening of the pelvis, and increasing the amount of body fat at the hips, thighs and bottom. It is also important for the growth of the uterus, development of the ovum and for normal menstruation.

> *Excess oestrogen may create deficiencies of zinc, magnesium and the B-vitamins, all of which are vital for hormonal balance.*

Oestrogen prepares the uterus for possible fertilisation and pregnancy every month, by developing an egg in the ovary and by thickening the lining of the uterus. Oestrogen is also critical for the normalcy of functions in a woman's body from digestion, to water and salt balance in blood and tissues, fat metabolism, health of the heart, blood vessels and bones.[27] It softens your cervix (mouth of the uterus). It helps produce vaginal secretions which both lubricate and aid the sperm in swimming well. The functions of this hormone are essential even for the health of our brain, as it has a huge impact on our memory and emotions.[28] An imbalance in oestrogen levels can be devastating for a woman's health due to the sheer magnitude of functions performed by this hormone in our body.

Oestrogen in PCOS

Women with PCOS often have oestrogen dominance. This can occur with high levels, or even with normal levels, of oestrogen. This 'dominance' is not in terms purely of the levels of oestrogen alone, but in comparison to the levels of the hormone progesterone. Oestrogen is said to be dominant when the ratio of progesterone to oestrogen is lower than ideal. According to Dr Lam, for optimum health, the progesterone to oestrogen ratio should be approximately 200 to 1. [29]

An absence of ovulation, as occurs in many women with PCOS, leads to a drop in progesterone levels (as progesterone is released after ovulation, from the corpus luteum). This shifts the ratio of oestrogen to progesterone towards one of oestrogen dominance.

In obese women with PCOS, their fat tissue can convert the free circulating testosterone to oestrogen. This surplus oestrogen contributes to higher levels of oestrogen, also creating an environment of 'oestrogen dominance'.[30]

Relatively high levels of oestrogen in PCOS can affect the feedback loop to certain parts of the brain (the hypothalamus and pituitary) and can alter the levels of Luteinising Hormone (LH) and Follicle Stimulating Hormone (FSH) levels. This can upset the menstrual cycle.[31]

Tell-tale signs of oestrogen dominance in PCOS[32]

- Infertility
- Absent or abnormal periods
- Severe PMS-like symptoms such as breast tenderness, headaches, mood swings, weight gain, water retention
- Decreased sex drive

- Fatigue
- Insomnia – difficulty falling and staying asleep
- Hair loss
- Decreased memory.

Dangers of oestrogen dominance

Oestrogen dominance can increase the risk of developing high blood pressure, breast cancer, endometrial cancer (cancer of the lining of the uterus), infertility, osteoporosis (brittle bones), stroke, diabetes and heart dis-ease.[33,34]

Tests to detect oestrogen dominance

Simple tests like a saliva test can be used to assess the levels of oestrogen, progesterone and many other hormones. These tests can be done at home and are easy, non-invasive, inexpensive and accurate.[35] Some of the latest 'Female hormone profile – capillary blood test kits' provide you with the freedom of testing your hormonal levels within the comfort of your home. They are simple, minimally invasive and accurate.[36] Your medical doctor or other health care professional can also refer you for these tests.

How to balance oestrogen levels?

To reduce the levels of oestrogen to within optimal levels, you need to reach your ideal weight, and improve your food plan and lifestyle. Here are some suggestions:

- Increasing your physical activity can help you lose weight and will thereby help to balance your oestrogen: progesterone balance.
- Healthy ways to manage stress, like Yoga and meditation will help you balance your oestrogen levels.
- Avoid the birth control pill – birth control pills often

contain synthetic oestrogen, adding to your oestrogen load and oestrogen to progesterone imbalance.

- Processed and refined foods need to be removed (or at least reduced). Processed and sugary foods include white bread, cake and bakery products.
- Eliminate, or reduce, alcohol consumption.[37]
- Eat plenty of fibre from fresh fruits, vegetables and some gluten-free whole grains.
- Indole-3 carbinol is a compound contained in cruciferous vegetables like broccoli, Brussels sprouts, cabbage and kale. It is essential for balancing oestrogen levels.
- Omega-3 fatty acids, such as those contained in flaxseeds, tofu, walnuts, olive oil and in fish like tuna, salmon, mackerel and swordfish, also help in restoring the oestrogen balance.[38]

Xenoestrogens

Chemicals such as parabens, commonly used as preservatives in foods, toothpastes, cosmetics, shampoos and many more products, act like oestrogens when they enter our body. Similarly, breakdown products of DDT, other insecticides, laboratory detergents, industrial surfactants, wood preservatives, dyes and plasticisers may contain Xenoestrogens. Artificial hormones can also enter our body through consumed meat, poultry and dairy products. Heating our food in plastic containers, or drinking from warm plastic bottles, can increase our xenoestrogen load, as can exposure to pesticides and fertilisers. These artificial oestrogens can upset our hormonal balance.[39]

Progesterone

Progesterone is secreted by the ovary after ovulation (from the corpus luteum), and by the placenta during pregnancy.

Progesterone is vital for normal menstruation and fertility. It helps the uterus to prepare a cosy and nurturing environment in anticipation of receiving a fertilised egg. It also prevents shedding of the endometrial lining after the fertilised egg embeds in the womb. In addition, it inhibits the contractions of the uterus. Progesterone is essential in maintaining a pregnancy. A drop in progesterone levels can cause a miscarriage. Progesterone is rightly dubbed the 'pregnancy hormone'.

Progesterone is an important precursor for the production of other hormones. It also helps to maintain healthy blood sugar levels, thyroid function and normal water balance[40], is a natural antidepressant and promotes normal sleep.

Progesterone in PCOS

Women with PCOS who do not ovulate have decreased levels of progesterone. Remember, you can have a period, but not ovulate. The corpus luteum is produced after ovulation, when the 'empty egg shell' becomes this gland. The corpus luteum produces progesterone. If no ovulation occurs, the corpus luteum is not produced, and so progesterone is not produced. Some progesterone is produced in the adrenal glands, but this is not sufficient for healthy levels of this important hormone. Lowered progesterone levels, even with normal oestrogen levels, cause an oestrogen dominant situation.

Tell-tale signs of low progesterone

- Hair loss
- Irregular periods
- Heavy and/or painful periods
- Unexplained infertility
- Inability to maintain a pregnancy

- Extreme mood swings, panic attacks and depression
- Headaches, including migraine – often cyclical
- Tender or lumpy breasts
- Bloating and weight gain
- Back pain
- Fatigue
- Excessive premenstrual food cravings especially for chocolates and sweets.

Tests to detect progesterone levels

The saliva test and the capillary blood test (as described for oestrogen) can also be used to ascertain progesterone levels. You can also be referred by your medical doctor or health care professional.

Balancing progesterone

PCOS-related low progesterone levels have been effectively treated using physiologic doses of progesterone. Doses of natural progesterone in various forms aim to improve the level of progesterone, especially during the luteal phase of your menstrual cycle. We will discuss your menstrual cycle, and the luteal phase, in Chapter 13 – 'Boost Your Fertility – Learn how to increase your chances of not only becoming pregnant, but carrying your healthy baby safely through to term.'

Such natural supplementation can be in the form of one or more of the following:

- Natural progesterone (in oral form)
- Natural progesterone skin cream
- *Vitex agnus-castus* (Chasteberry) (promotes the production of progesterone).

I would always err on the side of nature. Supplementation has been shown to be incredibly safe and effective. Skin creams applied to the inner thigh, under the arms and the chest are the most effective as the absorption is faster.[41] You may need to see your medical doctor regarding natural progesterone. Vitex can be purchased from your health care professional.

A wholesome food plan and physical activity to promote weight loss – where needed – of as little as five to 10%, is often effective in restoring ovulation and so boosting progesterone. Vitamin C, zinc and vitamin A are important in the production of progesterone. Foods like rockmelon, organic liver and eggs have more than one of these important nutrients. See also your special bonus report at *www.ConquerYourPCOSNaturally.com/BonusReports* for a list of which foods are high in what nutrients. There are reports that wild yam contains hormone-like compounds similar to our progesterone. These compounds may boost progesterone levels.

Luteinising Hormone (LH)

Produced by the pituitary gland at the base of the brain, luteinising hormone (LH) is an important hormone for normal menstruation and fertility. A surge in the level of LH during the menstrual cycle leads to ovulation.

The status of LH in PCOS

The production of oestrogen from the ovaries is stimulated by LH. The pituitary gland then produces a surge in LH, designed to bring about ovulation. Ovulation leaves an empty egg shell, which becomes the corpus luteum and then produces progesterone. High levels of LH are found in approximately 60% of women with PCOS.[42] An imbalance of hormones such as LH and FSH (follicle stimulating hormone) in PCOS may lead to the incomplete maturation of an egg, and a following lack of ovulation. The elevated LH stimulates luteinising of the cells around the follicle. This can produce more testosterone and upset the menstrual cycle.

Why are LH levels often higher in women with PCOS?

Gonadotropin Releasing Hormone (GnRH) is secreted by the brain (the hypothalamus), released in pulses at a particular frequency and amplitude. Normally, slow frequency release favours the secretion of FSH and high amplitude release favours the secretion of LH. This difference regulates the secretion of Gonadotropins (LH and FSH). In PCOS, GnRH is released more often and at increased amplitude than normal, which favours the secretion of more LH than FSH.

In a woman with PCOS, LH level of 18IU/L and FSH level of 6IU/L are a typical find. Although these figures are 'within normal range', they represent an elevated LH:FSH ratio, also known as a ratio of 3:1.*

(http://www.obgyn.net/ displayarticle.asp?page=/pcos/ articles/hormone_levels_sterling)

* Measurements vary during the menstrual cycle.

Consequences of high LH

High levels of LH cause an imbalance of the LH to FSH ratio, shifting it to the higher side. The ovaries respond to increased LH stimulation by producing more androgen than oestrogen. The most common symptom of high LH levels is menstrual irregularity.[43] The most dreaded side effect of high LH levels is infertility. Studies have shown that women with high LH are less likely to conceive despite artificial reproductive therapies like in-vitro fertilisation (IVF). To make matters worse, 65% of women with high LH levels are prone to early pregnancy loss[44,45] and higher recurrent miscarriage rates.[46]

How to test your LH levels

You can check your LH levels by using a urinary ovulation predictor kit (LH-kit), typically around the time ovulation is expected. Your doctor, and some other health care professionals, can also refer you for blood tests to measure your LH levels.

How to balance the LH levels

Research studies conducted in obese women with PCOS-related infertility found a low calorie diet for six weeks helped to lower their LH levels. This diet also helped to balance the LH to FSH levels, and helped them to lose weight.[47]

Follicle Stimulating Hormone (FSH)

Produced by the pituitary gland, FSH is responsible for stimulating the growth of ovarian follicles. It also helps choose one egg to mature each cycle.[48]

Women with PCOS may have low absolute or relative levels of FSH. This means the FSH level may be low according to its outright value, or may be considered 'within normal limits' according its outright value, but may be low when looking at the LH to FSH ratio. The LH:FSH ratio is important for fertility. Hypothyroidism, which is more common in women with PCOS, can also decrease FSH levels.

The FSH connection in PCOS

Women with PCOS may have low levels of FSH. The levels of FSH should normally peak during the early phase of the menstrual cycle and mid-cycle. However, due to the negative feedback resulting from high oestrogen levels, the pituitary gland lowers its production of FSH. This lowered FSH level results in both decreased maturation of the eggs and the maturation of one egg (normally) for release. These immature follicles are not as sensitive to FSH, and so degenerate. A chronically low FSH level is a main cause behind the poor development of eggs, and anovulation (absence of ovulation) in women with PCOS.[49]

Losing weight, if needed, can help you balance the LH:FSH ratio and boost your ovulation and fertility.

Prolactin

Prolactin is a hormone produced by the pituitary gland. Its function is to stimulate and support the production of breast milk. This is the hormone of pregnant and breastfeeding mums. However, this hormone has another function – it suppresses two main hormones that are needed for ovulation – FSH and GnRH (Gonadotropin Releasing Hormone). Now you know why breastfeeding is a natural contraceptive!

Prolactin in PCOS

Prolactin is great for breastfeeding women. However, when it comes to PCOS, this hormone may not make you produce a lot of breast milk but, it may ruin your menstrual cycle and ovulation. It also acts against the corpus luteum, resulting in decreased progesterone production. Up to 30% of women with PCOS have high prolactin levels.[50]

High levels of testosterone, oestrogen and Insulin Resistance in women with PCOS, interfere with the action of the hormone prolactin, which can significantly reduce milk production in these women during the post-delivery period.

Elevated prolactin stimulates the production of androgens from the adrenal gland, thereby aggravating PCOS. Moreover, elevated prolactin levels may sometimes be the presenting evidence of an underlying hypothyroidism, which is another potential aggravating factor of PCOS. Hyperprolactinemia also causes sexual dysfunction in women by increasing the risk of painful intercourse (dyspareunia), causing a loss of libido, and decreasing arousal and orgasm.

Tell-tale signs of increased prolactin[51]

- Irregular or absent periods
- Milky discharge from the breast
- Tender breasts
- Signs of excess testosterone – hirsutism, etc.

Certain medications, stress, and a tiny tumour of the pituitary gland called a prolactinoma are some other causes which can increase prolactin levels. The levels of prolactin can be measured by a blood test. The test results are more accurate if the samples are taken just after waking, or after a person has been quietly resting for 30 minutes, as the levels of prolactin vary with the level of activity.[52]

How to balance prolactin

Foods that are high in zinc and vitamin B6 like fish, shrimp, tuna, sunflower seeds, soybeans, pinto beans and gluten-free whole grains may help your body to naturally reduce high prolactin levels. *Vitex* (Chasteberry) may also help to balance abnormal prolactin levels.

Dehydroepiandrosterone (DHEA)

DHEA is a weak 'male' hormone secreted mainly by the adrenal glands, and in small amounts by the brain and the ovaries. It is synthesised from cholesterol. It is a prohormone, being a precursor molecule, from which oestrogen, androstenedione and testosterone are made. During puberty, DHEA facilitates the growth of armpit and pubic hair. DHEA also helps to maintain healthy cholesterol balance and helps in managing body weight. Also, DHEA has stress-relieving effects and is believed to be a hormone that gives you natural protection from depression.[53]

DHEA connection in PCOS

DHEA levels are found to be high in women suffering from PCOS. Insulin Resistance and high stress levels may cause excessive DHEA in PCOS sufferers.[54] Other causes, such as abnormalities and tumours of the adrenal glands, can also cause high DHEA levels and may need to be ruled out by appropriate testing.

DHEA has some properties that are similar to testosterone.[55] When you have high levels of DHEA, the signs and symptoms will be similar to those of high testosterone:

- Oily skin
- Acne
- Excessive body and facial hair
- Irritability.

Blood tests can determine your DHEA level.

How to balance DHEA levels

The first step to balancing DHEA is to address Insulin Resistance. Eating plenty of healthy fibre will improve your SHBG levels, which will bind excessive DHEA in your blood.

Adopt healthy stress management techniques to bring your cortisol hormone level under control. As the levels of cortisol reduce, so will the DHEA.[56]

Thyroid hormones and PCOS

Your thyroid is a butterfly-shaped organ present in front of the windpipe in the neck. Thyroid hormones (thyroxine T4 and triiodothyronine T3) are essential in regulating your metabolic rate. In PCOS, there is a higher incidence of poor thyroid function and thyroid autoimmune dis-ease.[57] The combination of low progesterone relative to normal/excessive oestrogen levels may stimulate the immune system to attack the thyroid gland (autoimmune thyroiditis or Hashimoto's thyroiditis), causing hypothyroidism. Hypothyroidism contributes to obesity, lipid abnormalities[58], menstrual disturbances, lowered FSH levels and is linked with diabetes[59,60], all of which in turn aggravate PCOS. It also increases the risk of death from all causes, including coronary heart dis-ease.[61]

In addition, hypothyroidism may inhibit SHBG synthesis, leading to increased levels of free (and so active) oestrogen and testosterone. Thyroid levels can be assessed by assessing free T3, free T4 and Thyroid Stimulating Hormone (TSH) levels, plus thyroid autoantibody levels in blood after overnight fasting.

Your thyroid gland is discussed in greater detail in Chapter 9 – 'Your Thyroid – How to boost your metabolism, have abundant energy and lose weight'.

Homocysteine

Homocysteine is a metabolite – a product of normal metabolism. It is used to build and maintain tissue. However, high levels are dangerous to our health. With higher levels, there is an increased risk of heart attack and cardiovascular dis-ease.[62] A study in the *Journal of the American Medical Association*[63] found moderately high levels of plasma homocysteine were associated with greater risk of heart attack. To reduce homocysteine to ideal levels requires vitamins B6, B12 and folic acid. These are involved in the process of 'breaking it down'. If a person is deficient in these vitamins – due to lack of intake, lack of absorption or taking a medication such a Metformin[64,65] which is known to decrease the levels of these vitamins – homocysteine levels can remain high. Metformin has been linked to increases in homocysteine levels.[66] Levels of homocysteine have been found to be higher in women with PCOS.[67]

How to balance your homocysteine level

Implement the changes discussed throughout this book. Plus, add vitamin B6, B12 and folic acid rich foods and supplements. See your bonus report at *www.conquerYourPCOSNaturally.com/ BonusReports* for a list of foods high in these vitamins.

Cholesterol

Cholesterol has been given an undeserved bad reputation by the media and in medical circles. Did you know, without cholesterol you wouldn't stay alive, let alone thrive? Cholesterol is needed in our cell walls. It plays a critical role in cellular communication and is important for energy production. It is important both structurally and functionally for our brain. As Dr Dingle states: "Cholesterol is the starting material of many essential chemicals including vitamin D, steroid hormones and the bile acids necessary for digestion".[68] It even helps the function of our happy hormone, serotonin, and is important for our immune system. High cholesterol has been linked to heart dis-ease. However, low levels of cholesterol are also harmful to our health[69], and increase 'all-cause mortality'[70] – that means death from all reasons. As a woman with PCOS, you are more likely to have dyslipidaemia – an imbalance in the lipids in the blood. Please do not jump to the dangerous conclusion that a cholesterol-lowering medication will do anything to either address the underlying condition manifesting itself with a cholesterol imbalance, or in any way extend your life span or improve your health. These medications can also have serious – and deadly – side effects.

Balancing and maintaining healthy cholesterol levels is best, and most safely, done by adopting a healthy lifestyle.

PCOS affects the balance of many of your hormones. As you

will learn throughout this book, the levels of one hormone are affected by those of other hormones. Your body is like an intricate web, one thread being influenced by another, nothing occurring in isolation. With knowledge and action, it is possible to balance your hormones and conquer your PCOS.

Can't get enough?

Go to *www.ConquerYourPCOSNaturally.com/ BonusReports* to grab your FREE bonuses.

As an additional bonus, you'll also receive Dr Rebecca's *'Conquer Your PCOS'* monthly newsletter for FREE. You'll discover even more PCOS advice, easy-to-apply practical tips, PCOS-friendly recipes, and become a *'Conquer Your PCOS'* VIP.

Act now and join us and the 'Conquer Your PCOS' community!

Also, follow Dr Rebecca at:

www.Facebook.com/ConquerYourPCOS
and
http://Twitter.com/ConquerPCOS

Chapter Four

Deficiencies In Your Food Plan And Lifestyle

What you're missing out on is causing you harm.

> *"To eat is a necessity, but to eat intelligently is an art!"*
>
> *Francois La Rochefaucauld, Writer*

Ideally, the food we eat should provide us with the raw materials needed to grow, heal and think, the energy needed to function, the vitamins and minerals needed to enable necessary body reactions to occur, and the other vital components essential for optimal health.

Food is a necessity for us to survive, but optimal nutrition is essential for us to thrive. Although there is a surplus of food for the peoples of western nations, most humans suffer from deficiencies of various vitamins, minerals and other micronutrients.

More than two billion people (i.e. one in three) worldwide suffer from a deficiency of vitamins, minerals and other micronutrients.[1] This is not confined only to third world countries or the poor.

It is incredibly important for women with PCOS to overcome dietary deficiencies. Nutrients are essential for life and are required for each bodily process. These are required for correct insulin sensitivity, balanced and happy hormones, optimal brain function, a healthy gut and the list goes on. Pregnancy and lactation necessitates a higher demand for nutrients. Deficiency of vital nutrients in these crucial phases of life can jeopardise the health and even the life of your baby.[2]

Link between PCOS and dietary deficiencies

Our hormones, enzymes and every system in our body depend on the availability of nutrients. The status of micronutrients in your body will determine your fertility, and the outcome of fertility treatments if needed, and your weight loss efforts. Naturally, in one way or another, nutritional deficiencies lay the foundation of major dis-eases including PCOS.

Focusing on nutrition and removing deficiency is extremely important in conquering your PCOS. There are many factors that contribute to nutritional deficiencies:

- Exposure to environmental toxins
- Poor eating habits, extreme dieting, fad diets
- Poor digestion
- Food allergies and intolerances
- Long standing illness
- Certain medications
- Stress.

Your relationship with deficiency

The saga of nutritional deficiencies begins even before we are born. Poor maternal nutrition during pregnancy and breastfeeding can lead to increased risk of PCOS and obesity in a female child.[3]

Dietary deficiencies during adolescence can delay sexual maturation (delay in starting menstruation and in the development of reproductive organs), and increase the risk of early abortions and birth defects in future pregnancies.[4]

Insulin Resistance, a major driver in PCOS, is linked to several nutrient deficiencies. Recent studies have shown deficiencies in chromium, vanadium, zinc, vitamin D and carnitine can cause Insulin Resistance in both men and women.[5]

> ## *Girls versus boys:*
>
> *Teenage girls are more likely than boys to have low dietary intakes of vital nutrients. Dietary deficiencies at this crucial age of development set the stage for many diseases like PCOS, obesity, heart disease and diabetes!*
>
> Women and Health, *Marlene B. Goldman, Maureen Hatch, Gulf Professional Publishing, 2000, p279.*

Dietary deficiencies can contribute to obesity. Obesity can interfere with conception and lead to poor production of eggs and hormonal imbalances. This contributes towards infertility in women.[6]

The need to supplement

The nutrients in our food come from the soil and sun. As our modern day soils are deficient, so our foods are deficient also. To meet your nutritional needs, you must both eat well and supplement. Numerous research studies across the globe have proven the safety and efficacy of supplements. Any argument otherwise is simply born out of ignorance and incorrect information.

Make sure you choose high quality, potent supplements to ensure maximum absorption, reliability, results and great health.

Six key nutrients

Nutrition is an essential component in overcoming your PCOS. There are a number of nutrients you may be deficient in. Here, we will discuss six nutrients important specifically for improving insulin sensitivity, hormonal balance and essential to conquering your PCOS.

These key nutrients are often found to be deficient in women who suffer from PCOS, and we will shortly discuss some ways you can overcome these deficiencies.

1.   Chromium

Chromium is the 'shovel that puts fuel in the furnace'.

Chromium is an important component of the 'glucose tolerant factor' aka GTF (others being niacin, glycin, glutamic acid and cysteine). Chromium helps insulin in transporting glucose (sugar) from our blood into our cells. It also helps insulin to bind with the cell membrane. The levels of this element in our blood show direct effects on our insulin sensitivity and our blood glucose levels. No wonder chromium deficiency results in Insulin Resistance and glucose intolerance.[7]

Chromium is crucial for keeping blood sugar levels stable and reduces food cravings. Research studies have found that

> ## How much chromium do you need?
>
> *Daily supplements of 400–600mcg of chromium are safe and well suited for people who are Insulin Resistant.*
>
> *Chromium is better absorbed when taken as chromium picolinate.*
>
> Natural Supplements for Diabetes: Practical and Proven Health Suggestions for Types 1 and 2 Diabetes, *Frank Murray, Len Saputo, Basic Health Publications, Inc., 2007, p113.*

chromium reduces excessive food intake.[8] Also, it is found to be lower the higher the levels of insulin in the blood – commonly seen in Insulin Resistance.[9] By improving insulin sensitivity and decreasing the cravings for carbohydrates, chromium helps in weight loss.[10] Indulging in sweet, carbohydrate rich food, refined flour products and processed foods strips our body of chromium. Meanwhile, eating complex carbs helps in preserving it.[11]

Foods rich in chromium are white fish, fresh parsley, olives, whole grains, spinach, mushroom, ripe tomatoes, raw onion and romaine lettuce.

2.   Magnesium

Magnesium is required for more than 300 enzymatic reactions in our body. The latest statistics reveal up to 40% of the American population gets less than 75% of the Daily Value of Magnesium.[12] Remember also, daily values (or Recommended Daily Intakes – [RDIs]) are a bare minimum to avoid a dis-ease – not what is required to achieve true wellness. Magnesium deficiency has been reported in areas ranging from Australian and New Zealand livestock, to Egyptian children and pregnant women in India.[13]

Like chromium, magnesium is important for the transport of glucose across the cell membrane and insulin sensitivity. Harvard

How much magnesium do you need?

Daily supplements of 300–400mg of magnesium are recommended.

It is best to take magnesium along with calcium supplements for better absorption.

Natural Supplements for Diabetes: Practical and Proven Health Suggestions for Types 1 and 2 Diabetes, *Frank Murray, Len Saputo, Basic Health Publications, Inc., 2007, p122,* Stop Diabetes Now: A Groundbreaking Program for Controlling Your Disease and Staying Healthy, *(Google eBook), by William T. Cefalu, Penguin, 2009.*

researchers found a correlation between lower magnesium intake and a higher risk of diabetes.[14] Magnesium is also vital for energy production in the liver.[15]

Insulin Resistance, heart dis-ease, depression, PMS, high blood pressure, and pre-eclampsia, to name only a few conditions, have been linked to low levels of magnesium; *www.mgwater.com* is a good resource.

Insulin Resistant people, such as those with diabetes and PCOS, are found to have low magnesium levels. Women with metabolic syndrome and systemic inflammation (again, common in PCOS – see Chapter 7 'Oxidative Stress – What is it, why it can kill you, and how to defeat this fertility assassin') also suffer from low magnesium levels.[16] Studies show that women with PCOS have significantly lower serum levels of magnesium.[17]

Food sources of magnesium are oats, rice bran, dried coriander, chives, nuts, spinach, flaxseed oil, sunflower seeds, fruits such as passionfruit, bananas, blackberries and raspberries, and dark chocolate.

3.   B vitamins

The B vitamin family is a very important nutrient group for women with PCOS:

- Vitamin B1 is crucial for carbohydrate metabolism.
- Vitamin B2 helps in conversion of fat, sugar and protein into energy.
- Vitamin B3 helps to keep blood sugar levels in balance, and is a component of glucose tolerance factor (GTF). It also helps make sex hormones, lowers LDL and increases HDL, helping to maintain healthy cholesterol levels.
- Vitamin B5 helps in controlling fat metabolism and, hence, helps weight loss.

- Vitamin B6 is necessary in maintaining hormonal balance, and normal metabolism. It is also important in brain function and glucose tolerance.

B vitamins stabilise our appetite and improve digestion, particularly of carbohydrates. Their deficiency leads to poor carbohydrate digestion, which can result in abnormally high blood glucose levels. An Australian study showed diabetics – who have similar levels of Insulin Resistance to women with PCOS – were deficient in B vitamins, particularly in Vitamin B6.[18]

> *How much B complex vitamins should you take?*
>
> *Take a good B complex supplement that contains at least 50mg of each of the major B vitamins.*
>
> *It is better to take B complex supplements than taking individual B vitamins.*
>
> Smart Medicine for Healthier Living: A Practical A-To-Z Reference to Natural and Conventional Treatments for Adults, *by Janet Zand, Allan N. Spreen, James B. LaValle, Penguin, 1999, p499.*

An imbalance of B vitamins, especially vitamin B2, is associated with an abnormality in oestrogen and progesterone levels leading to menstrual irregularities and even infertility.[19]

In Chapter 6 'Stress – Learn how to beat stress, rediscover happiness, regain your focus and get your mojo back', I discuss further the links between stress and the hormonal imbalance of PCOS. B vitamins are revered as 'anti-stress' vitamins due to their stress-lowering effects. This makes B vitamin supplementation and an increase in vitamin B rich foods very important for women with PCOS.[20]

Some of the common signs of B vitamin deficiency are lowered stamina, getting tired easily, loss of appetite, irritability, poor memory and emotional instability.[21]

Gluten-free whole grains like quinoa, amaranth, buckwheat and brown rice contain good amounts of B vitamins. Nuts, legumes, eggs, green leafy vegetables and fish are also rich sources of B vitamins.[22]

4.   Zinc

Zinc is an important mineral with "a clear role in the synthesis, storage and secretion of insulin".[23] High levels of blood glucose due to the Insulin Resistance in diabetes and PCOS can cause a high loss of zinc from the body. Apart from being important in the correct functioning of our insulin, zinc is an antioxidant and anti-inflammatory.[24] These benefits are an absolute necessity when you have PCOS.

> ## How much zinc do you need?
>
> *A daily dose of 25mg of zinc supplement is a minimum.*
>
> *It is best to take copper supplements along with zinc since zinc has a tendency to mobilise copper out of the body.*
>
> Dietary Supplements and Functional Foods, *(Google eBook), by Geoffrey P. Webb, Wiley-Blackwell, 2006, p106.*

Zinc deficiency can result in reduced fertility and increased risk of miscarriages[25] and can cause growth retardation in babies, premature delivery, low birth weight babies and delivery complications.[26]

Research studies have found that heart dis-ease, diabetes and glucose intolerance are significantly higher in those who ingest lower amounts of zinc. Also, people who are obese are more likely to have abnormally low levels of zinc.[27]

Signs and symptoms of a zinc deficiency include acne[28], white spots or lines across the fingernails[29], painful periods (dysmenorrhoea)[30], altered taste, impaired wound healing[31], and possibly inflammatory bowel dis-ease.[32]

Organic lean meat, fish and poultry are rich sources of zinc.

Oysters are one of the best seafood sources of zinc.[33] Plant sources include avocado, spinach, mushroom, pine nuts, pumpkin and sesame seeds, beans, nuts, and garlic.

5.   Co enzyme Q10

Co enzyme Q10 (CoQ10) is essential for energy production and as an antioxidant offering protection from harmful free radicals. Women with PCOS are known to have low antioxidant levels. CoQ10 also plays an essential role in protecting your cardiovascular system – including your heart.[34] CoQ10 improves your body's ability to produce energy, and may help to reduce Insulin Resistance.

Natural sources of CoQ10 include eggs, spinach and broccoli, and fish such as mackerel and sardines.

Cholesterol lowering statin drugs cause CoQ10 deficiency

Use of statin drugs are known to cause CoQ10 deficiency. Women with PCOS often have an imbalance of lipoproteins – the cholesterol-carrying proteins – in their blood. These women are often prescribed statin drugs with the misguided belief this will in some way prevent health complications such as heart dis-ease. However, although cholesterol-lowering drugs do 'drop the numbers', they do not extend life or address the underlying cause. These medications are used to 'normalise' cholesterol readings, but this does not correlate to improved health. As Professor Dingle states in his 2009 November Newsletter, cardiovascular disease (CVD) "is not a disease of cholesterol or even cholesterol accumulation… Cholesterol is associated with the risk of CVD but it is not the disease".[35] Statin drugs deplete our levels of co enzyme Q10. This can cause muscle aches, cramping and weakness. These drugs also cause infections, suicide, cancer and more. For more information on statin drugs, please read the free secret special reports included with this book: *Putting Statins in Perspective* and *Dr Dingle's Newsletter*. (Go to *www. ConquerYourPCOSNaturally. com/BonusReports*. It will be delivered to you as a secret bonus!)

> ## How much CoQ10 do you need?
>
> *A daily dose of 50mg of CoQ10 as ubiquinol (which is a more active reduced form of ubiquinone).*
>
> *CoQ10 supplements work best when taken before your cardio exercises or interval training sessions.*
>
> *Also, taking CoQ10 with healthy fat-containing foods – like almonds – assists with optimal absorption.*
>
> The Fat-Burning Bible: 28 Days of Foods, Supplements, and Workouts that Help You Lose Weight, *by Mackie Shilstone, John Wiley & Sons, 2004, p106.*

6.   Omega-3 fats

In western society, our food plans tend to include a great deal more omega-6 than omega-3 fatty acids. This imbalance leads to inflammation. American diets, for example, tend to contain 14–25 times more omega-6 than omega-3.[36] Omega-3 fatty acids are crucial to our health. I cannot overstate this. Increased omega-3 fat intake has been shown to reduce serum triglyceride levels, blood pressure and cardiovascular dis-ease. It even protects the heart from damage following a heart attack and the brain from damage following a stroke. It stabilises cell membranes, has anti-inflammatory properties[37], helps cell communication[38], improves mood[39] and improves insulin sensitivity.[40] For a woman with PCOS, omega-3 fatty acids are essential to a healthy, happy, PCOS free life.

Signs and symptoms of omega-3 deficiency include fatigue, poor memory, depression[41], period pain, infertility and postpartum depression.[42]

Sources of omega-3 fatty acids include cold water oily fish such as salmon, herring, anchovies and sardines, fish oil, krill oil, green lipped mussels, chia seeds, flaxseed oil, walnuts and walnut oil, and microalgae.

NOTE: Some people cannot convert vegetarian sources of omega-3 into the DHA noted to have important health effects.

Modern farming practices and nutritional deficiencies

Modern farming methods have radically changed the nutrients available in our food. Pesticides, fertilisers and animal pharmaceuticals are now frequently used.

Let's compare

A comparison was conducted between the quality of eggs produced by hens grown on free-range farms and those from hens raised indoors on a factory farm. This revealed the free-range eggs contained up to 30% more vitamin E, 50% more folic acid and 40% more vitamin B12 than the eggs of factory-raised hens.[43]

Facts about the plummeting nutritional values of common foods[44,45,46]:

- Potatoes appear to have lost 47% of their copper content, 45% of their iron and 35% of their calcium in the period ranging from 1940 to 1991.

- Calcium content of broccoli averaged 12.9 milligrams per gram of dry weight in 1950. In 2003, the figure stood at 4.4mg/g dry weight.

- The average vegetable found in the supermarket today is at least 5–40% lower in minerals including magnesium, calcium, zinc and iron than those of 50 years ago.

- Protein concentrations declined by 30–50% between the years 1938 to 1990.

Depletion of the minerals in our soils is also alarming.

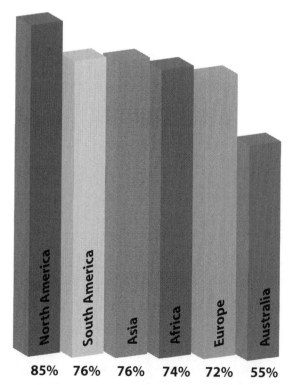

Percentage of mineral depletion from soil during the past 100 years, by continent.

Source: www.tjclark.com. au/colloidal-minerals-library/soil-depletion.htm

North America	South America	Asia	Africa	Europe	Australia
85%	76%	76%	74%	72%	55%

Anti-nutrients

> "*Optimum nutrition is not about what you eat – what you do not eat is equally important!*"
>
> Patrick Holford, author, The New Optimum Nutrition Bible

Anti-nutrients are chemicals, mostly man-made, in our food. The two attributes needed for qualification as an anti-nutrient are:[47]

1. Their presence in our food stops nutrients from being absorbed by our intestines, and/or;

2. Their presence in our food and body promotes the excretion of nutrients from our body.

Going organic:

The best way to ensure wholesome nutrition without the negative effects of anti-nutrients is to choose organic foods, where possible. Some benefits include:

- *It's tastier, healthier and more nutritious*
- *It's environmentally friendly*
- *Better for animal welfare*
- *Absence of genetically modified content*
- *Minimisation of toxins including pesticides, fungicides and xenoestrogens.*

Needless to say, anti-nutrients need to be avoided to ensure optimum nutrition.

Some major anti-nutrients you need to watch for are:

1. Genetically modified organism (GMO)

A genetically modified organism (GMO) is an organism (animal and plant alike) whose genetic material has been modified using genetic engineering techniques. GMO foods are altered to grow bigger, yield larger harvests, to be herbicide tolerant and insect resistant. Common GMO foods include soy, corn, potatoes, cottonseed, canola oil and zucchini.

We do not yet know the full extent of the effects of GMO foods. However, one study conducted on 20-week-old mice fed with GMO corn revealed this group had greatly impaired fertility as compared to mice fed non-GMO corn.[48] Reports of a Russian study showing hamsters fed GMO soya beans had slower growth rates, slowed sexual maturity rates and sterility, should have us concerned.[49]

2.   Pesticides, herbicides, antibiotics and hormones

Chemicals sprayed on to our food, or fed to our livestock (hormones and antibiotics are fed to poultry and farm animals), can impact on human fertility. Exposure to harmful chemicals can add xenoestrogens, and negatively impact hormonal balance, thyroid function and even the central nervous system.

3.   Specific foods

Some common foods and drinks are anti-nutrients.

- Alcohol
- Refined sugar
- Hydrogenated fats and oils
- Water from plastic bottles.

4.   The toxic jungle of food colours, additives and preservatives

Ten per cent of what we eat in everyday life is not actually food, but a toxic brew of additives, colours and preservatives. These additives act as anti-nutrients and deplete the nutritional value of our foods. Artificial food colours may be derived from petrochemicals and tar, neither of which are fit for human consumption.

Read food labels carefully. Any ingredient lists you can't pronounce, and any 'food' with a long list of non-food sounding ingredients are best left on the shelf.

Watch for the following food additives, as apart from depleting the nutrient content of your food, they may cause a series of health complaints:[50]

- Butylated Hydroxyanisole (BHA) and Butylated Hydroxytoluene (BHT)
- Propyl Gallate
- Sodium Nitrate/Sodium Nitrite
- Sulfites (Sulfur Dioxide, Sodium Sulfite, Sodium and Potassium Bisulfite, Sodium and Potassium Metabisulfite)
- Potassium Bromate
- FD&C Blue No. 1
- FD&C Blue No. 2
- FD&C Green No. 3
- FD&C Red No. 3 (Erythrosine)
- FD&C Yellow No. 5 (Tartrazine)
- FD&C Yellow No. 6
- Monosodium Glutamate (MSG)
- Acesulfame-K.

Poor food habits

Fad diets, junk food and poor food choices cause nutritional deficiencies. Low calorie and very low calorie diets cause water and nutrient loss from the body. A stressful lifestyle can place upon you greater nutritional demands, leading to nutrient deficits.[51]

Common signs of nutrient deficiencies

Knowing the basic signs and symptoms of nutrient deficiencies is a good place to start. Refer to the chart below for insight into possible deficiencies.

Common signs and symptoms of nutrient deficiencies:

NAME OF NUTRIENT	KEY SIGNS
CALCIUM	Brittle nails, depression, insomnia, irritability, osteoporosis, palpitations, tooth decay, delusions, loss of muscle tone, muscle cramps
POTASSIUM	Muscle weakness, tiredness, water retention, vomiting, low blood pressure, continual thirst, poor kidney function
IRON	Anaemia, tiredness, brittle nails, confusion, depression, constipation, dizziness, fatigue, headaches, mouth lesions, inflamed tongue
OMEGA-3 – FATTY ACIDS	Mood swings, depression, memory loss and neurological problems
VITAMIN A	Acne, dry hair, growth impairment, fatigue, insomnia, weight loss, night blindness, thickening and roughness of skin
VITAMIN B	Indigestion, chronic fatigue, nervousness, constant uneasiness, frustration, rashes, tingling in hands, soreness
VITAMIN C	Bleeding gums, depression, joint pains, easy bruising, loose teeth
VITAMIN D	Burning sensation in mouth, insomnia, nervousness, muscle cramps, weakness, tingling
CHROMIUM	Fatigue, glucose intolerance, anxiety
COPPER	Anaemia, fatigue, diarrhoea, hair loss, fragile bones, weakness
ESSENTIAL FATTY ACIDS	Dry skin, diarrhoea, hair loss, acne, gall stones, PMS, poor wound healing, infertility
FOLIC ACID	Diarrhoea, headaches, insomnia, paranoia, weakness, breathlessness
IODINE	Fatigue, weight gain, hypothyroidism
MAGNESIUM	Anxiety, confusion, insomnia, heart attack, irritability, restlessness, weakness, cramping
ZINC	Acne, amnesia, brittle nails with white spots, growth impairment, hair loss, high cholesterol levels, irritability, loss of sense of taste, impotence, depression, diarrhoea

Deficiency beyond your food plan

Due to the significant role factors like stress play in your health, and maybe even in the development of PCOS, yet another 'deficiency' needs to be given a thought. Deficiency of positive thought is not an uncommon feature in women suffering from PCOS. Infertility, a quality of life less than wished for, fear about the future, and feeling inferior and self-conscious about body image are some major factors pushing women with PCOS to think negatively.[52] Repeated failure at conceiving and repeated miscarriage, as well as what may seem like an impossible path to weight loss or clear skin, can also add to negativity.

Your state of mind and your thoughts affect your entire body. It can alter your hormonal balance, change your hunger patterns and impact on your digestion. Your thoughts are an important part of your health. Negative thoughts (and a scarcity of positive thinking) pose a major roadblock in your crusade against PCOS.

It is very important to boost positive emotions, positive self-image, positive thinking. To do this, you may need to change your beliefs. This is not just so you 'feel better'. Your thoughts literally change your biology.

Stress management, meditation, positive affirmations, counselling and energy balancing techniques like Yoga, Tai Chi, and Qigong are priceless tools when it comes to increasing positive beliefs and so positive emotions. You may find joining a PCOS support group valuable. These groups provide you with a platform to openly express your feelings, to share experiences and to feel a sense of belonging. Isolation breeds negativity.

Support from your loved ones, friends, peers and family is also crucial for boosting positive emotion and reducing negativity. For more information on improving and involving your loved ones, read and have them read, Chapter 16 'Communicate Well – A guide for your loved ones to understand and support you.'

Deficiency also includes deficiency in movement. Movement of particularly your spinal joints, but also the other joints in your body, literally energises your brain. With a deficiency in movement – the major nutrient for your brain – you can neither be well, nor conquer your PCOS. This requires correct segmental movement (through Chiropractic) and movement of the body as a whole (physical activity). For more information on improving your brain function through movement, read Chapter 11 'The Magic Of Movement – How to simply and easily incorporate movement into your life. Plus, I reveal the single training tip for quicker, easier fat loss and hormonal control.'

Deficiency in sleep is also a significant problem. Lack of sleep decreases insulin sensitivity, and so can escalate PCOS and the symptoms that come with it. Women with PCOS are also more likely to suffer from sleep apnoea.

Can't get enough?

Go to *www.ConquerYourPCOSNaturally.com/ BonusReports* to grab your FREE bonuses.

As an additional bonus, you'll also receive Dr Rebecca's *'Conquer Your PCOS'* monthly newsletter for FREE. You'll discover even more PCOS advice, easy-to-apply practical tips, PCOS-friendly recipes, and become a *'Conquer Your PCOS'* VIP.

Act now and join us and the 'Conquer Your PCOS' community!

Also, follow Dr Rebecca at:

www.Facebook.com/ConquerYourPCOS
and
http://Twitter.com/ConquerPCOS

Chapter Five

Your Gut

Learn how to stop that embarrassing wind, relieve your bloatedness and tummy pain, and improve your PCOS.

> *"All disease begins in the gut."*
> *Hippocrates (460–377 BC)*

Your gut is incredibly important for your health. It transports, breaks down, absorbs, detoxifies and protects. Hippocrates really was a man before his time, in his appreciation of just how important our gut is to our well-being.

When you eat, the food is initially placed in your mouth. Here begins the process of breaking down (chewing and wetting) and digesting (by digestive enzymes in saliva) foods. Then you swallow. This muscle contraction pushes the food into your food pipe (your oesophagus) and then into your stomach. A healthy working stomach produces just the right amount of acid to further break down the food you have eaten. From here, it travels into your small intestine. Your small intestine breaks down the food further, and absorbs nutrients and water from the eaten food. From here, it goes through your large intestine and finally out through your anus.

Through the gut, there can be areas that work sub-optimally. This can have a significant impact on your health.

Digestive enzymes are important in breaking down the food eaten. Each type of the three main food types (macronutrients) – carbohydrate, protein and fat – requires different enzymes to break them down. If you have less than optimal digestive enzymes, you can't effectively break down the food. This in turn means you can't absorb its goodness.

TIP: A tablespoon of organic apple cider vinegar just before a meal can help with proper digestion.

Your small intestine is very important to your health. I will focus on it somewhat, as not only does it have the important job of breaking down the food further, and absorbing nutrients, it also houses some incredibly important bugs called your microbiota.

Think of your small intestine like a hole in a doughnut; the inside of your intestine is really like the outside of you. In a healthy gut, the lining of the small intestine determines what gets through into your body. This lining can be damaged, or become 'leaky' (known medically as 'increased intestinal permeability', or 'translocation'), and our gut can become inflamed. When this happens, endotoxins, hormones, food particles, and parts of bacteria and yeast can pass through into our body. We can develop an inability to correctly absorb nutrients, and to stop things that shouldn't get through into our body, passing through.

So, how is this relevant to PCOS?

Well, before we get started, let's quickly define some terms.

Definitions:

Inflammation: Is the way a body responds to being hurt. Inflammation is swelling in your body's tissues; sometimes it causes pain and redness. Inflamed tissue contains damaged cells and increased blood flow – which is why it's red and warm. It is often 'infiltrated' by immune cells/healing cells (see *www.science. org.au/nobel/2005/glossary.htm*).

Bad bugs: Bacteria in our gut which are harmful to us. They may be bacteria, fungi, viruses or yeast that are not meant to be present, or ones that are normally present – but are in too greater numbers.

Endotoxin: A part of bacteria that is toxic in our bodies.

Endotoxemia: The presence of endotoxins in the blood.

Now...

Women with PCOS may have an increased rate of Irritable Bowel Syndrome[1] and also have increased levels of inflammation.[2,3] A leaky gut can increase systemic inflammation.

Women with PCOS often suffer from oestrogen dominance. Excessive oestrogen in our body should be bound, and so inactivated. An enzyme called beta-glucuronidase breaks down the bound oestrogen in our gut destined for excretion. This now free oestrogen can now be resorbed, and further increase oestrogen levels. This enzyme can be formed by the 'bad bugs' in our gut, especially when they are higher in numbers than ideal. On top of this, increased oestrogen can increase the growth of yeast *(Candida albicans)*[4] in our gut. Increased yeast can increase leaky gut, thus causing more inflammation, more bowel symptoms, decreased gut function, decreased nutrient absorption, and the possibility of greater oestrogen absorption.

Leaky gut can be caused by an imbalance of the bacteria in your intestine, deficiencies in the immune system, and increased leaking through or damage to the gut wall.

Leaky gut is promoted by:

• Endotoxemia

- Starvation
- An increase in the bad bugs (intestinal dysbiosis, or overgrowth). This condition can be caused by oral antibiotics. Antibiotics are often overprescribed, and sometimes used in women with PCOS to treat acne.[5]

Women with PCOS may have a higher incidence of bulimia.[6] Bulimia causes health issues, and can lead to deficiencies in the nutrients important for maintaining the health of the gut, such as zinc, L-Glutamine, and vitamin A.

In each human, there are approximately 10 trillion human cells. There are also 90 trillion gut bugs, called microbiota. This means you are actually nine-tenths gut bugs! Rather than thinking of us as us, and the gut bugs as gut bugs, it is more accurate to think of us as a living, thriving city. We are the building, the bugs are the inhabitants. The good bugs are the nurses, the policemen, the chefs, the builders. The bad bugs are the criminals and the riff raff. As long as there are enough good bugs to protect, to monitor and to heal, order is maintained. Your good gut bugs perform many important functions for your body's metabolism and immunity. They keep the bad bugs in check, produce vitamins necessary for good health, and provide defence against external threats.

Q: Why are our gut bugs (probiotics), and the food that feeds them (prebiotics), important in PCOS and for our general well-being?

Cutting edge research shows:

- Probiotics reduce obesity caused by a high fat diet, Insulin Resistance, glucose intolerance and fatty liver.[7]
- Probiotics decrease body weight.[8,9]
- Probiotics and prebiotics may decrease inflammation, and improve your immune response.[10] Given inflammation

is a driver in metabolic syndrome – and PCOS – this is particularly relevant.

- Prebiotics reduce body weight gain and fat mass development.[11]
- Prebiotics lower food intake and body weight.[12]
- Fatty liver dis-ease (NAFLD) occurs at a higher than normal rate in women with PCOS.[13,14] A leaky gut places more stress on the liver to detoxify harmful substances. Prebiotics have been shown to improve a fatty liver, and a leaky gut.[15]
- Prebiotics improve insulin sensitivity, and decrease liver glucose production.[16]
- Prebiotics decrease liver inflammation.
- Two great bugs for the health of gut are called Bifidobacterium and Lactobacillus. Prebiotics increase both these bugs.[17] A high fat diet decreases the numbers of Bifidobacterium.[18]
- Prebiotics reduce plasma lipids.[19]
- Prebiotics reduce a leaky gut.[20]
- Prebiotics decrease systemic and liver inflammation and oxidative stress.[21]
- Prebiotics improve insulin signalling.
- Prebiotics increase the feeling of 'fullness', decrease the feeling of hunger, reduce the food eaten and help control blood sugar levels.[22]

So, the bugs in your gut really are important in human health, especially for a woman with PCOS.

You now have some insight into the importance of our good gut bugs and the food that feeds them. The prebiotics are dietary fibres. I strongly recommend increasing the foods in your food plan containing these pre and probiotics (see the free report at *www.*

ConquerYourPCOSNaturally.com/BonusReports). In our modern day environment, which is successful in killing our good gut bugs and increasing our bad gut bugs, I highly recommend regularly taking a high quality probiotic supplement. The probiotic should contain bacteria indigenous to humans, organisms that resist degradation by acid and bile, be packaged in a dark container, be refrigerated, and contain species shown to have positive health effects in therapeutic doses. Your health care specialist will be able to guide you further.

NOTE: I do not recommend the liquid brands laced with sugar.

Now, a little more about leaky gut...

The vicious cycle of a leaky gut (Leaky Gut Syndrome or LGS)

Factors that may have contributed to a leaky gut initially – like obesity – are then worsened by the development of LGS.

Rapid commercialisation has drastically increased our exposure to toxins and chemicals. Our bodies continue to face the challenge of protecting us from the toxins we are exposed to, whether these come from our environment, food, or personal and cleaning products. When working well, the human body has special pathways to remove most toxins which we come into contact with.

The passage of food

At least two-thirds of your immune system lies within your gut.

From the time you place food into your mouth, to the time it reaches your colon, your body is busy digesting, processing and separating healthy nutrients from undesirable toxins.

As you eat, the food enters your digestive tract – basically one long tube from your mouth, through the oesophagus, stomach and small intestine, then finally to your colon, and out.

Let's talk more about your small intestine, an amazing part of your body, the lining of which is only one cell thick.

It has two important functions:

- To absorb nutrients; and
- To act as a barrier to toxins, bad bugs and large food particles.

The lining of your intestine performs the all-important function of selectively allowing in those nutrients required, and keeping out those things we don't need, or that can hurt us. Any damage to this lining affects its ability as a barrier, and can allow substances that shouldn't pass through, to pass through into the body.

Most mainstream medical practitioners do not recognise, or know about, Leaky Gut Syndrome. Medications are often used in an attempt to treat each of its symptoms separately. However, your gut can only be restored to health when the items causing harm are removed and the damage is repaired. Removing toxicity and supplying the nutrients required for healing and health are the only way to overcome a leaky gut.

Leaky gut – the process

The spaces between the small cells lining your gut (epithelial cells) become wider than normal. This allows the passage of harmful particles through your intestinal lining, and into your bloodstream. Harmful particles include the likes of toxins, parasites, fungi, bacteria, yeast, undigested proteins and food particles. In simpler terms, the wall of your gut should act like a funnel to harmful products. In leaky gut, it is more like a sieve.

Once a toxin passes through the lining of your gut, your immune system swings into action. Your body begins the process of defending itself from 'the foreign invader'. Inflammation and irritation result. As leading international nutrition expert Dr Jeffrey Bland states: "leaky gut triggers a state of continuous and prolonged stress in and on the immune system". This can affect not only your gut, but also your whole body. And as your body fights, it produces 'free radicals' and increases your need for antioxidants. We'll learn later in Chapter 7 'Oxidative Stress – What is it, why it can kill you, and how to defeat this fertility assassin' that women with PCOS are already low in antioxidants. The ramifications of this are profound for your health now and into the future.

PCOS and the need to detox

Leaky gut syndrome (LGS) can cause pain and discomfort, dis-ease and embarrassment. It can also cause inflammation throughout the body, hormonal disruption, an increase in our toxic load, and an inability to properly absorb the nourishment we need from our food and drink.

What can we do about LGS?

Firstly, you need to improve your food plan. Give your body what it needs to be healthy. Stop eating those things that stress your gut. These not only cause damage, but require many nutrients to repair the damage they cause. Our bodies like foods that are easily digestible (natural). We also need non-digestible food components, such as insoluble fibre. Insoluble fibre feeds and keeps our good gut bugs happy and healthy.

Let's have a look at our body's own natural detoxification system and what happens when it fails to handle toxic overload. The excretory system of the human body functions through seven of its key organs and fluids, including:

- Skin
- Blood
- Liver
- Kidneys
- Colon
- Lymph
- Lungs.

Each of these organs plays its own vital role in relieving the body of metabolic waste and environmental toxins. Failure of this mechanism due to any factor impairs the functioning of the body and damages its tissues and cells. This may eventually lead to major system failures.

The need for detoxification is heightened in our modern day life. When our body's delicate mechanisms of self-detoxification fail or function sub-optimally, we become ill. We do not function as we should. A leaky gut requires a detoxification and cleansing program.

The PCOS link

By definition, detoxification is a process of eliminating poisonous or toxic substances from the body. It neutralises the effects toxins play on the body and allows healing to take place.

When planning a PCOS detox, remember the following:

- *Keep your fruit consumption limited to lower-GI carbs, including the likes of apples, oranges, peaches, plums, grapefruit and grapes.*
- *Make sure you consume healthy proteins with each meal.*
- *Eat cruciferous vegetables such as broccoli, cauliflower, cabbage, bok choy, Brussels sprouts etc.*
- *Add turmeric and cinnamon to your food.*
- *Drink a lot of pure water (but don't drink from water in plastic containers).*

In women with PCOS, detoxification is important. And the best food plan for a woman with PCOS is not dissimilar to that required for detoxification; i.e. low GI carbs along with lean protein sources, as nature intended, and preferably organic.

In addition, if you do not repair your gut lining and overcome a leaky gut, you are likely to suffer from nutritional deficiencies. This will aggravate your PCOS. Take the case of magnesium. Low levels of magnesium are linked with insulin resistance. Deficiencies in this mineral will exacerbate PCOS. Or low zinc levels. Low zinc levels will affect the optimal functioning of important hormones such as insulin, and zinc is essential in repair, and for fertility.

NOTE: Muscle cramps, period pain, high blood pressure and constipation can occur with a magnesium deficiency.

NOTE: White spots under your fingernails can indicate a zinc deficiency.

You can expect to achieve the following benefits from a well-structured, professionally guided, detoxification program:

- Better digestion
- Clearer skin
- Improved energy levels
- A clearer, less foggy, mind
- Weight loss
- A happier, more balanced mood
- Enhanced sleep
- Less muscle and joint pain
- Improved immune function.

LGS and obesity

Our gut is equipped with an incredibly important component

of our immune system. When problems such as a weakening of your gut lining occur, this directly impacts on your immune system function. Toxicity and inflammation occur, and these two conditions are known to lead to obesity.

The process

When you are suffering from a leaky gut, toxins that are ordinarily kept from entering your body – by your gut – can pass through. They can then proceed, with the products of the inflammatory response they cause, into your blood stream. Once there, these toxins produce inflammation throughout the body, contributing to obesity (see below).

Leaky gut syndrome and obesity

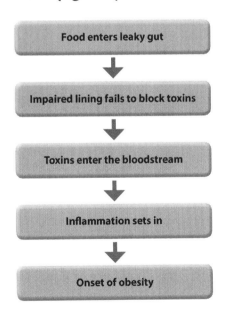

There is much research linking high levels of inflammation with obesity and excessive weight gain. One such study compared a marker of inflammation (the level of high-sensitivity C-reactive protein [CRP]) in overweight children and those who were of normal weight. The overweight kids had a three-fold higher CRP level than the normal weight kids.[23]

The links between obesity and Leaky Gut Syndrome have been established in groundbreaking research conducted by Patrice D. Cani. With his team, the effects a change in gut bugs (microbiota) caused on inflammatory levels in obese mice were studied.[24,25,26]

They clearly established that obese and diabetic mice displayed increased intestinal permeability i.e. a leaky gut, metabolic endotoxaemia and low grade inflammation.[27] Feeding these mice with prebiotics increased the number of intestinal bifidobacteria (good gut bugs) and reduced the impact of high fat diet-induced metabolic endotoxaemia and inflammatory disorders.[28,29] The type and number of gut bugs may be significantly different between healthy and obese individuals.[30]

Hormonal influences

One of the key functions of our liver is to break down the unused hormones and send them off for removal from our body via the gut. However, in the case of LGS, the liver is already overloaded. It becomes less effective at removing excess hormones and other toxins. Without the removal of these substances, they build up in our body.

A leaky gut can impair the body's ability to remove toxins and excess hormones from the body. Let's look at oestrogen. Oestrogen is a vital hormone in the body. However, an excess of this hormone can cause health challenges. We are exposed to oestrogenic chemicals in our environment, our food and our drink. Many women with PCOS also have higher relative levels of oestrogen. This increase in oestrogen needs to be addressed, and removed from the body. When we have a leaky gut, we have less ability to remove excessive levels of oestrogen. The body removes 'used' oestrogen and oestrogen compounds by a process known as glucuronidation. Glucuronidation allows these 'used' hormones to be inactivated (by being bound) and excreted through the urine or faeces.

One mechanism that allows the body to maintain its oestrogen balance — by removing excessive amounts of this hormone — can be disrupted by an enzyme known as beta-glucuronidase.

Enzymes that act in the same fashion, with the same results, as beta-glucuronidase come from 'bad gut bugs' (such as *Escherichia coli*). This enzyme 'frees up' the bound oestrogen. This now free, and active, oestrogen can be resorbed into the body, particularly when you have Leaky Gut Syndrome, and exert its oestrogenic affects once more. Interestingly, glucuronidation is the same process by which many commonly prescribed drugs and food ingredients are detoxified, including the likes of aspirin, menthol, vanillin (synthetic vanilla), food additives such as benzoates, and some other hormones. Experts point out the healing properties of calcium d-glucarate (CDG), which is a natural ingredient found in certain fruits and vegetables (like apples, grapefruit and broccoli). It is believed CDG can reduce the action of beta-glucuronidase and facilitate the elimination of oestrogen, and other toxins.

Your thyroid gland is another organ that bears the impact of poor gut health. You can read more about the thyroid gland in Chapter 9 'Your Thyroid – How to boost your metabolism, have abundant energy and lose weight'. A leaky gut may contribute to the development of hypothyroidism, and autoimmune dis-ease. T4 (a thyroid hormone) may also be affected by the enzyme beta-glucuronidase, in the same way as it affects oestrogen.

Food intolerances

As LGS is in big part caused by food habits, and the way your body responds to what you eat and drink, it comes as little surprise that this condition is associated with a series of food intolerances (most common), as well as food allergies.

As we read earlier, a leaky gut allows incompletely digested food particles to cross the gut barrier. Our body then identifies these as *foreign invaders*. This triggers off an immune response, and can further damage your gut lining.

The most common food intolerances and allergies are:

- Dairy protein, called casein (cow's milk, cheese, cottage cheese, yoghurt, ice cream)
- Gluten grains (wheat, rye, spelt, barley)
- Beans (soy)
- Almonds
- Peanuts
- Eggs (if you are not intolerant, I must point out eggs are a super food!).

The two food groups that contribute most to intolerances are gluten and dairy. Although I do not recommend milk, limited dairy such as yoghurt on a rotation basis is often well handled. I cannot in good conscience recommend any person eat gluten, ever.

Gluten, a protein found in foods such as wheat and barley, can cause Coeliac dis-ease, reportedly affecting about one in a hundred North Americans. However, I want you to know that you can be Coeliac free, but still intolerant to gluten. Gluten to a person with coeliac dis-ease is a poison – one portion of gluten can cause inflammation of their gut for approximately three months. To a non-coeliac, gluten intolerant person, the reaction is not as dramatic. However, it does have significant adverse health effects that need to be addressed. When Professor Loren Cordain was asked how to tell if someone is gluten intolerant, he looked at his audience and simply asked 'are they human?' This would be my response also. We have deliberately increased the gluten present in our grains from 4%, to 17% (for increased shelf life). Add to this all the products gluten is sneakily added to, and you have a large daily dose of this toxin.

NOTE: The consumption of gluten is associated with an increased production of zonulin, a protein capable of increasing the intestinal permeability in humans as well as animals.[31] If you eat meat, consider what happens when you consume the products of animals fed gluten.

Meanwhile, for dairy products, the main cause of intolerance is casein, a milk protein.

TIP: When these dairy and gluten products enter our bodies, they can produce products known as *casomorphines* and *glutomorphines...* which as the name suggests cause an addiction. Have you noticed those people who just can't live without milk or bread?

Checklist for optimal gut health

* Take your time while eating.
* Focus on what you are eating.
* Eat where you can relax (not at your desk, on the run etc. This takes your focus away from digestion).
* Do not eat in front of the TV (watching negative images such as the news may stress your body, and stress and digestion are not optimally compatible).
* Chew thoroughly – this begins mechanically breaking down your food, and begins digestion.
* Eat foods congruent to health promotion; i.e. organic vegetables, organic meats and fish.
* Consume foods high in the nutrients beneficial to optimal gut health; i.e. Zinc (see your bonus report on 'What If The Food Already In Your Cupboard Could Help You Conquer Your PCOS?' at *www.ConquerYourPCOSNaturally.com/ BonusReports)*
* Avoid processed, unnatural foods. If your great-grandparents wouldn't recognise it as food, chances are your body can't either. There are modern day

'foods' that not only provide no nutrition, but also take nutrients from your body to break them down. These include 'foods' from well-known fast food establishments, foods with artificial flavours, preservatives and other additives, and foods high in sugar. For more information, see Chapter 4 'Deficiencies in your food plan and lifestyle – What you are missing out on is causing you harm' and specifically the information on *anti-nutrients.* Better these are not part of your food plan.

- Avoid foods that you are intolerant to, the most common being gluten and dairy.
- Regularly take a high quality pre and probiotic.
- Drink enough pure water.
- Better manage your stress.
- Exercise regularly.
- Get enough magnesium-rich foods.
- Eat foods rich in good fats; i.e. fish, avocado, nuts and eggs.

Can't get enough?

Go to *www.ConquerYourPCOSNaturally.com/ BonusReports* to grab your FREE bonuses.

As an additional bonus, you'll also receive Dr Rebecca's *'Conquer Your PCOS'* monthly newsletter for FREE. You'll discover even more PCOS advice, easy-to-apply practical tips, PCOS-friendly recipes, and become a *'Conquer Your PCOS'* VIP.

Act now and join us and the 'Conquer Your PCOS' community!

Also, follow Dr Rebecca at:

www.Facebook.com/ConquerYourPCOS
and
http://Twitter.com/ConquerPCOS

Chapter Six

Stress

Learn how to beat stress, rediscover happiness, regain your focus and get your mojo back

> *"Every stress leaves an indelible scar, and the organism pays for its survival after a stressful situation by becoming a little older."*
>
> *Dr Hans Selye*

These words of Dr Hans Selye – a pioneer in identifying the hazardous effects of stress – are prophetic. Stress is a double-edged sword. It is our saviour in times of peril and our worst enemy in our pursuit of health. Some amount of stress is good; it keeps our bodies finely tuned and adaptable. However, when stress becomes significant or chronic, when it pushes you towards distress, the saga of stress-related adaptation (you may think of this as 'disease') unfolds. Dr Selye was the father of the famous theory of 'General Adaptation Syndrome', which explains how chronic exposure to stress depletes health and leads to dis-ease.[1] He believed more than the factors which cause stress, it is the way we respond to these stressors that lead to dis-ease. Ongoing research has proven his theory correct.

Women are three times more likely than men to suffer from disorders like depression in response to stress. Also, women often experience much stress in their personal and professional lives. This increases the risk for many disorders, like PCOS.[2]

How and where does stress fit in with PCOS?

Stress and PCOS share a complex relationship. In simple words, we can say that these two have a hormonal bond. The hormonal changes our body undergoes while adapting to prolonged stress and those changes found in women suffering from PCOS are strikingly similar.[5]

Stress works hand in hand with other factors. The genetic information in your recipe book of life, and environmental and lifestyle factors contribute to the development of PCOS. You may be shocked to know that the stress-related hormonal changes that can contribute towards PCOS are seen even in girls who are still in their mother's womb. Various research studies done in this field point to chronic stress as a cause, complicator and intensifier of the symptoms of PCOS.[6]

Uncertainty about the progress and meaning of this syndrome, failure to see results with previous care, and the social stigma attached to various symptoms of PCOS again serve as a recipe for increased stress in a woman with PCOS.

1. The tale of stress and PCOS

Modern lifestyle has 'bullied' us. We consider ongoing stress as a part of normal, daily life. However, the effects of stress go much deeper than frazzled nerves or an occasional dropping of the bundle. Stress influences almost every aspect of PCOS.

Hysterical hormones

We women know that stress can imbalance our hormones, and affect our mood. Stress can cause, as well as exacerbate, the hormonal imbalance of PCOS.

Cortisol

Cortisol is a key stress hormone, and links stress and PCOS. Cortisol gives us that burst of energy for the 'fight or flight' response. This hormone is designed for release when we are faced with an acute, life-threatening situation – like being attacked by a predator. Once the attack ends, our cortisol levels should reduce back to optimal levels. However, the constant stress we are often faced with in modern life means the figurative attack doesn't end. This can cause chronic excessive levels of cortisol in the body. This results in a snowball effect, creating one hormonal imbalance after another. These compounding changes may produce the symptoms of PCOS.

Insulin, hormones of the hypothalamus and pituitary glands and hormones of the ovaries are some of the major hormones that are affected by excess cortisol. According to Dr David Zava, biochemist, researcher and author, "excess cortisol keeps our hormones from operating at optimal levels."[7]

Women under chronically high levels of stress are unable to deal with stress effectively. High stress levels cause your body to switch into life-preservation mode. You stop thinking clearly, and may feel scattered. You can look for the escape paths, but you can't add simple arithmetic. Your memory is affected. You can become self-focused. You are 'geared up for the fight' and live on edge, white-knuckled and unable to relax. Your blood pressure and pulse rate rise. Your immune system and reproductive function lowers. Your bone formation decreases. Your body and brain are simply trying to survive the threat they believe you are under. These changes occur to divert your blood and energy to only the functions required for a successful flight or fight. You run the programs necessary for survival. This takes energy away from the systems not required at that exact moment in time, like becoming pregnant, writing your shopping list, healing a wound or digesting your food. You are surviving, not thriving. To add to the misery of PCOS, excessive cortisol can then be converted into male hormones.[8]

Insulin Resistance: Excess cortisol generated by stress makes the body cells resistant and unresponsive to the hormone insulin. Thinking about this in a survival situation, it is an intelligent decision for your body to make. If insulin cannot draw the glucose into your cells, it remains in your bloodstream – ready to fuel your escape from the imminent threat. However, chronic Insulin Resistance is deadly. Insulin Resistance is a serious problem for your health, and a significant cause of PCOS and the symptoms that occur as a result of it.

Insulin Resistance means our cells are unable to appropriately absorb glucose. This literally starves the cells of glucose and leaves you feeling tired.

Stress can cause women to choose sweet tasting, and fatty food and drink over more healthy options, and can lead to emotional eating and bingeing. Stress can compel you to make a beeline for the refrigerator, pantry or supermarket junk food aisle. The sugary and fatty foods allow your body the energy it needs to continue the fight. The effects of stress are worst in those women who eat in an attempt to cope with stress.[9]

Approximately 80% of women suffering from PCOS have Insulin Resistance. Almost 95% of women with obesity, with or without PCOS, have this metabolic problem.[10]

High levels of insulin in the blood coax the ovaries to produce more male hormones, or androgens. An excess of male hormones like testosterone are a hallmark sign of PCOS.[11]

Insulin Resistance can lead to life threatening conditions in women with PCOS. In fact, it is an underlying reason for many lifestyle dis-eases such as diabetes and cancer. Insulin Resistance increases low density lipoprotein (LDL) in the blood, and increases the risk of hypertension, stroke and heart dis-ease.[12]

Obesity around your middle: Insulin Resistance causes your body to store excess fat – leading to weight gain and obesity. Obesity in PCOS is seen particularly around the thighs, hips and the middle of the body, over the abdomen (aka 'central adiposity'). Insulin Resistance creates major road blocks to the process of losing weight. Obesity is known to aggravate Insulin Resistance, which starts yet another vicious cycle of obesity and Insulin Resistance.[13] Insulin Resistance also reduces levels of another hormone called 'leptin', which controls the expression of hunger. An imbalance of leptin can lead to erratic eating habits.[14]

Hairy issues: Losing scalp hair and the abnormal growth of thick facial and body hair, are yet further distressing symptoms suffered by women with PCOS. The hormone that links stress with these symptoms of PCOS is pregnenolone. Pregnenolone is produced when we get stressed. This hormone is needed for cortisol production and helps us cope with stress.[15] Excessive pregnenolone however causes a series of hormonal changes, such as the excessive production of male hormones. This in turn causes classic symptoms of PCOS like the development of 'cysts' in the ovaries, and increased levels of male hormones leading to acne, loss of scalp hair and excessive facial hair.[16]

Another way stress can contribute to PCOS is by reducing the levels of Sex Hormone Binding Globulin (SHBG). One of the functions of SHBG is to inactivate excessive testosterone in the blood. The levels of SHBG dwindle in women who suffer from prolonged stress. This leads to an increase in the levels of free testosterone in the blood.[17] Testosterone triggers the unwanted hair growth, loss of scalp hair and acne suffered by many women with PCOS.

Infertility: Stress can cause abnormalities in the hormones of the hypothalamus and pituitary, leading to an imbalance of the female reproductive system. Abnormally high levels of male hormone prevent the growth and maturation of the eggs in the ovaries and leads to 'cystic ovaries'. Stress strains the thyroid gland, reducing the level of follicle stimulating hormone (FSH). The resulting hormonal imbalance reduces the maturation of an egg, leading to cystic ovaries, anovulatory cycles (menstruation without producing an egg)[18], irregular cycles, or potentially no cycles at all.

Eighty to 100% of women suffering from PCOS have disorders of ovulation and 33–75% of women with PCOS suffer from infertility.[19]

If your brain and your body think you are in a fight for your life (stress), it makes complete sense not to divert energy into creating a baby. You need that energy now, or you won't survive. Making babies can be left for another day, at a safer time and place. The problem is, most modern day stressful situations are not life threatening, they are just perceived this way by our body and brain. Fertility problems arise when this safer time does not come.

The emotional side of PCOS: PCOS may push a woman toward the abyss of depression, anxiety, and low self-esteem, and can degrade her quality of life. The long journey toward a confirmed diagnosis, weight gain, unwanted hair growth, acne, infertility, irregular periods, and the uncertainty of PCOS can make even the toughest cookie crumble. Stress in this case is both the cause and effect. It triggers the hormonal imbalances that cause PCOS and the symptoms of PCOS in turn create more stress. The psychological impact of PCOS in women is largely underestimated and often ignored.[20]

Normally, an acute stress is followed by the release of our

happy hormone, serotonin. This magical hormone calms down our nervous system and body, and reduces our stress response. When we are under chronic stress, our serotonin levels become depleted. We cannot replenish this critical hormone as needed, and we essentially run out of the amount required to return us to a healthy state. It's like trying to continually scoop water from a gushing, leaky bucket. We then become depressed, tired and grumpy. We lose our sex drive, which compounds our inability to become pregnant (after all, no sex is a great guarantor of no baby). We don't sleep well, which affects our ability to lose weight and have the energy and motivation to move. This makes us even more grumpy, and more stressed. The cycle continues...

TIP: Movement increases serotonin. See Chapter 11 'The Magic Of Movement – How to simply and easily incorporate movement into your life. Plus, I reveal the single training tip for quicker, easier fat loss and hormonal control' for ways to easily increase your movement.

2.   Managing stress the right way

PCOS is still a poorly understood syndrome. Our current understanding of this dis-ease may be just the 'tip of the iceberg'. Many health care providers lack any real understanding, so you may find yourself trawling the internet, praying for answers. They can be very hard to find. As PCOS is a syndrome, a combination of many appropriate responses to an inappropriately toxic and deficient environment and lifestyle, no pill can fix it. If you are advised a pill is the answer... please, please do yourself a favour – run a mile. Nor can a simplistic approach to dealing with a single symptom help you truly overcome your PCOS. Our bodies work like a web, intricate and interrelated. One part of your journey to success over PCOS is managing your stress. This is necessary to overcoming any, and all, of your symptoms and in conquering this syndrome.

Stress can diminish your ability to effectively adopt health promoting food choices and required movement. These are vital in overcoming your PCOS. Hence, choosing great ways to manage stress is a most important step towards conquering your PCOS. Although stress is a major contributor to PCOS, to its pathogenesis and perpetuation, its importance is significantly under-recognised by conventional society. Unless the 'stress factor' in PCOS is addressed, attempts at conquering your PCOS may fall short. This may well be the piece of the puzzle you are missing. I cannot emphasise this enough.

Conventional therapies utilise synthetic agents, foreign and toxic to your body, to merely suppress a symptom. They interfere with one pathway, without regard to the other processes they affect. They can cause side effects that can be as serious as the syndrome itself. This doesn't address the underlying cause of your syndrome, the whys of your body's adaptive behaviour. And they add a higher stress burden to your body.

Chronic stress affects your mind and body, as well as your spirit. A holistic approach to address stress is required. Holistic therapies emphasise healing and restoring health by revitalising and strengthening a person's innate healing abilities. As a Chiropractor, my job is simply to remove interference to your nervous system, so your body can heal and function as it should. Not to presume I am the one doing the healing for you, or that I know better than your cells what your body needs. This is the necessary approach. To my mind, it is the only approach. After all, your body, given sufficiency and purity, will do amazing things and produce the incredible health you deserve.

By the way, lifestyle and 'alternative' therapy has been scientifically proven to trump drug therapy in the treatment of metabolic syndrome *every time!*

3. Holistic therapies for stress management

There are various holistic therapies that are beneficial in helping you cope with stress. However, it should be understood that stress management is not a one-day gig, it is a lifetime commitment. These therapies require dedication on your part. You need to just 'keep at it'. Remember, it took your body years to get to where it is now. It will take time to reverse the damage, and a lifetime to maintain your balance on the life/stress see-saw. You would maintain a brand new Ferrari, and your body is worth infinitely more than a car. As my mum once said, "anything worth achieving takes time and effort". Trust me, it's worth it.

You've got to move!

Women with PCOS are more prone to depression, which is a major stress on the body and brain. Professor Irwin Kirsch's research showed psychotherapy and exercise outdoors are more effective than antidepressants for helping depression.

So, what kind of physical activity?

Yoga: When it comes to managing stress, Yoga is incredibly empowering. A branch of Yoga called Hatha Yoga is well suited to relieving stress and boosting health and vitality. It leads us to our natural stress-free state through a series of body poses or 'asana', breathing exercises or 'pranayama' and meditation or 'dhyana'. Yoga is especially beneficial for women with PCOS. Iyengar Yoga is my favourite type of Yoga.

Yogic exercises, breathing and meditation techniques help our body cope with stress by reducing stress hormones such as cortisol. Yoga practice has been found to be beneficial in women suffering from anxiety and depression.[21] Also, Yoga helps to balance the function of endocrine glands like the hypothalamus and the pituitary gland, which is crucial for the health of the reproductive system.[22] Yoga teaches us to look beyond our physical appearance and to embrace our amazing body. Good Yoga practices should be learnt from a trained professional and should be tailored to a person's body type and condition.

T'ai Chi: T'ai Chi is a form of martial art that uses slow, flowing and calculated movements to increase body balance, awareness and flexibility. T'ai Chi is often dubbed 'moving meditation'. Just like Yoga, T'ai Chi helps to reduce stress by directly lowering the stress hormone – cortisol. The practice of T'ai Chi boosts positive emotion, enhances vigour and reduces anxiety.[23] T'ai Chi is easy to learn and its regular practice can work wonders for you.

Qigong: Qigong (pronounced 'chi kung') is a term used for various Chinese energy exercises and healing practices. Qigong involves a series of slow-moving meditations and integrated mind-body exercises for enhancing and nurturing our vital energies. This therapy is not just time tested, but its effectiveness has also been proven through scientific research. Qigong can be a real boon to women who suffer from stress and PCOS. Qigong helps us to cope with stress by increasing our 'happy hormones' – our endorphins – which help us to feel relaxed and joyful. It reduces stress hormones like cortisol and brings balance to other hormones in the body.[24] Qigong is fast being recognised as an effective solution for stress management.

Just remember, though, any movement is good. If you love it, do it. Don't forget to also add incidental movement to your day. Incidental movement is unstructured movement. Take the stairs instead of the escalator. Sweep instead of vacuum. Walk at golf instead of using the buggy.

What else?

Acupuncture: Acupuncture is a Chinese healing science that involves the stimulation of specific points on the body to improve specific body functions, relieve dis-ease and promote health. Acupuncture has been used for centuries, and is especially useful for relieving pain and emotional stress. Acupuncture uses the insertion of fine surgical needles by a trained professional at specific body points. Believe it or not, the whole procedure is less painful then tweezing your eyebrows. Some Acupuncture therapists also use a newer version called electro-acupuncture.

Acupuncture can relieve stress, as well as the symptoms of PCOS. It reduces stress hormones, and helps us cope better with stress. It also pampers us by increasing our happy hormones – leaving us relaxed and refreshed.[25] The effects of acupuncture can be long-lasting. It is an ideal therapy for a woman with PCOS because of its fertility-enhancing abilities. Acupuncture helps in development of normal eggs in the ovaries, thus improving your chances of having a baby.[26] Research has also shown it to be effective in improving insulin sensitivity.

Chiropractic: Dr Roger Sperry, M.D (Nobel Prize Recipient for Brain Research) discovered "90% of the stimulation and nutrition to the brain is generated by the movement of the spine". Without correct spinal motion, joint sense (proprioception) and mechanical stimulation (mechanoreception) is decreased, while harmful, or noxious, input (nociception) is increased. This faulty input into your brain causes decreased brain function. As your brain coordinates every cell in your body, this has serious repercussions on your health. This is where Chiropractic comes into its own. Chiropractic care normalises the movement of your spine. A recent study has shown that Chiropractic adjustments improve brain function.[27] Chiropractors give prime importance to your spine, as your spine is integral to the function of your nervous system. The spine not only supports the pathway through which the nervous system carries impulses to and from our body and brain, it is a very part of this system. Chronic stress and poor segmental spinal movement both cause nerve irritation, decreased brain function, muscle tension and a raft of other changes in your body.

Chiropractors know that a healthy and well-balanced spine is a key in successful stress management. Specific spinal adjustments performed by your Chiropractor also reduce the muscle tension often associated with stress[28] and relax your body and mind. Chiropractic care helps your brain to step down from the 'fight or flight' mode.[29] Three of the most common responses I hear in clinic are: "I feel so much better in myself", "I feel less grumpy" and "I've noticed I'm sleeping much better since I've started care". It's amazing what can happen when your body and brain are able to communicate correctly.

Aromatherapy: Aromatherapy uses the sense of smell to promote healing. Our sense of smell shares a very intimate relation with our emotions, thoughts and overall well-being. I'm sure you've experienced the lift a specific scent can bring to your mood, or the memory that floods back from long ago. Aromatherapy may be beneficial in relieving stress Aromatherapy is the perfect way to pamper yourself and boost your health at the same time.

Aromatherapy uses essential oils of various herbs and flowers for inhalation, massage or for bathing purposes. Aromatherapists will usually prepare a synergistic blend of various essential oils, depending on your body type and symptoms. The essential oils that are commonly used for relieving stress and specifically for symptoms of PCOS are: Jasmine, Geranium, Clary Sage,

Lavender, Ylang Ylang, Chamomile, Bergamot, Cedar, Rose and Sandalwood.[30] You can use oils for self-massage (dilute the essential oil in a few drops in olive oil or vegetable oil) or add a few drops to your bath water for a luxurious soak.

Massage: Massage uses the hands to ease muscular tension, break adhesions and improve blood flow. It is wonderful in the promotion of health, for enhancing function, in helping your body's detoxification processes, and for promoting relaxation and well-being. It is a wonderful way to decrease both your physical and emotional stress.

Naturopathy: Naturopaths encourage optimal nutrition and use other therapies and remedies to help you cope with stress. The deficiency of certain nutrients can significantly contribute to stress. The cravings, emotional eating, crash diets and altered hunger patterns commonly associated with stress and PCOS can lead to nutrient deficiencies.

Naturopaths encourage healthy eating habits, use specific supplementation and introduce lifestyle changes for optimal health. Regular mealtimes and improved eating habits help digestion and efficient absorption of nutrients. A wholesome food plan including a variety of foods such as fresh organic fruits, vegetables, gluten-free whole grains, nuts, seeds, fish and controlled portions of poultry and lean meats, will give you immense nutritional benefits. If it wasn't for the healing science, ancient wisdom and cutting edge research of Naturopathy, much of the nutrition knowledge we now have would be severely lacking. This amazing profession, along with Chiropractic, is pushing research ahead, and carving out a path towards true wellness. In your quest to both reduce your stress – and to conquer your PCOS – you need both a Chiropractor and Naturopath standing supportively in your corner.

What about supplementation?

If your body is mineral or vitamin deficient, replacing these lost nutrients is essential to your well-being. There are certain nutrients that are critical to your sanity, too.

What supplements can help you de-stress?

A good old multivitamin supplement will help by providing a little amount of many nutrients. Supplements containing zinc, magnesium, coenzyme Q10, B vitamins and omega-3 not only help in rectifying the metabolic changes associated with PCOS, they are also great at reducing stress levels.

'Theanine' is an inexpensive supplement you can buy over-the-counter. It is also a nutrient found in green and black tea. Theanine helps to calm your mind, and increases mental sharpness and alertness.[31] Theanine supplements can be taken in a dose of 50 to 200mg daily on a regular basis, or when you are in need of some relaxation.

Overindulgence in certain foods can increase your stress levels. I need to tell you, caffeine is one such culprit. Although caffeine can lift our mood briefly, excessive tea or coffee can actually have the same effect as long-term stress. If you are addicted to tea or coffee, it is better to taper down your consumption rather than stopping it suddenly.

Alcohol is another substance women with PCOS should be wary of. Alcohol can increase stress hormones and cause anxiety, lack of sleep and nervousness. It can also contribute to obesity, a leaky gut and adds a toxic burden to your body.

Most processed foods and fast foods are crammed with sugar and salt to please your taste buds. The more we have, the more we want. For some women, one bite of a sugar-filled food will lead to another and another. You may be left with the guilt of a failed diet, another uncontrolled binge, and an empty cookie jar. Sugar adds significantly to the stress placed on your body and mind. It may also increase negative emotions like worry, fear and melancholy. If you want to claim back your peace of mind and banish excessive stress from your life, go easy on the basics like sugar.[32]

These are ways you can decrease your stress levels, even in these busy times. Implement small changes to start – remember to take some deep breaths, sing loudly while dancing to your favourite tune, dance naked (in privacy is probably best!), eat a beautiful raspberry while fully focusing on the taste and texture, say an affirmation regularly, don't watch the news, drink more pure water, get enough sleep, receive regular Chiropractic care. These activities don't eat up a lot of time from your day. Then, as you become accustomed to new practices, maybe take a Yoga class, consult a health professional for a more tailored approach, enjoy a holiday. Plan your day – with rest and periods of physical activity included. Not only will this change your life and attitude over time, and help you conquer your PCOS and increase your fertility, it will also decrease your chances of suffering one of the biggest killers in our society like heart dis-ease, stroke, cancer – all at least partially stress related.

Can't get enough?

Go to *www.ConquerYourPCOSNaturally.com/ BonusReports* to grab your FREE bonuses.

As an additional bonus, you'll also receive Dr Rebecca's *'Conquer Your PCOS'* monthly newsletter for FREE. You'll discover even more PCOS advice, easy-to-apply practical tips, PCOS-friendly recipes, and become a *'Conquer Your PCOS'* VIP.

Act now and join us and the 'Conquer Your PCOS' community!

Also, follow Dr Rebecca at:

www.Facebook.com/ConquerYourPCOS
and
http://Twitter.com/ConquerPCOS

Chapter Seven

Oxidative Stress

*What is it, why it can kill you, and
how to defeat this fertility assassin*

What is oxidative stress?

You will have heard how important it is to include a lot of fruits and vegetables in your food plan. Perhaps you have heard it's important to take supplemental antioxidants. Maybe you have heard about 'super antioxidants', 'super foods' or supplements that promise to make you look and feel younger. Our global society is full of advertisements – but short on explanations. In this chapter, you will learn why antioxidants – both natural and the supplemental variety – are so important.

In nearly all of the essential biochemical reactions occurring in our bodies, there are transfers of electrons (negatively charged particles). When an electron, with its negative charge, is transferred to a molecule, that molecule is said to be 'REDuced' – because it becomes more negative. When a substance loses an electron, it becomes more positive, and is referred to as being 'OXidised'. This category of biochemical reaction is called a REDOX reaction and is happening constantly in every cell of our body. These reactions occur predominantly in our mitochondria. The mitochondria are featured in many basic biology classes as the 'powerhouse' or the 'battery packs' of the cells. The function of the mitochondria is to release the energy found in foods in a form that our cells can use – these functions come under the category of cellular respiration – in other words, this is how our cells 'breathe'.

During these redox reactions, by-products are produced called 'free radicals'. A free radical has one extra electron (unpaired electron) and that makes it *very* unstable and *very* reactive. There are various types of free radicals – there are the Reactive Oxygen Species (ROS) and the Reactive Nitrogen Species (RNS) and others. Perhaps, you've heard the phrase "nature abhors a vacuum"? Well, nature doesn't much like an unpaired electron either, and that is why free radicals are so unstable. They need to 'grab' an electron – and they *will* from any nearby molecule. This is what causes damage, as a free radical will grab an electron from DNA, a nearby protein or lipid/fatty acid... or anything else it can. In the process of grabbing the electron, the free radical damages the DNA, the protein or the lipid/fatty acid, and that damages the cells, the tissues and the organs. The mitochondria can be particularly damaged as so many redox reactions take place there. When enough mitochondria become damaged, there is a decrease in the amount of energy produced, and even more damage results. The 'powerhouse' has been switched off – there's no more 'juice' in the battery.

It is the build-up of this oxidative stress that we call 'inflammation'. Our bodies have a great ability to compensate and repair the damage, but eventually we (and our cells) can't compensate anymore, and the levels of inflammation in our body increase. The oxidative stress our cells and tissues undergo can, in the end, result in a large number of different dis-eases – including PCOS[1,2,3], heart dis-ease[4,5,6], diabetes[7,8,9], metabolic syndrome[10,11], infertility[12,13,14,15], and obesity.[16,17,18] Which condition you may develop depends on many factors, including your 'book of life' (your genes), your exposure to various toxins, any deficiencies, stress, and how active you are (or aren't). It is important to remember that free radicals DO perform vital functions in the body – in killing off viruses and bacteria, in the immune response and in cell communication.[19,20,21] On the down side, free radicals are thought to be involved in the aging process. One theory proposes that aging is the accumulation of the damaging effects of free radicals.[22,23]

While the production of free radicals is a natural and at times even advantageous process, when excessive it can become a *serious* problem. Nature, as it tends to do, provides a natural control mechanism for reducing free radical damage.

There are a number of systems, called antioxidant systems, designed to limit and 'mop up' free radical damage. Some of the most important antioxidants naturally found in the body are glutathione, CoQ10, vitamins A, C and E, niacin, ferritin and the trace mineral selenium.[24] In addition, the omega-3 fats in fish oils are wonderful in protecting against the damaging effects of free radicals, and in reducing inflammation. Under healthy conditions, these natural antioxidants help prevent just the sort of damage described earlier. Even more impressive is the fact that many of these natural antioxidants can be efficiently recycled.[25,26,27,28,29,30] However, while these natural antioxidants can be recycled, they can also be overwhelmed by free radicals, particularly once the inflammatory process has set in.

Our environment contains many toxins, heavy metals and man-made synthetic substances which promote oxidation and are known to be pro-inflammatory (cause inflammation).[31,32] For example, among the cells of the immune system there are cells that, when exposed to toxins in the air, tend to favour a pro-inflammatory response. If these types of immune cells are stimulated often enough, asthma may result.[33] Fat cells tend to promote inflammation – being overweight can essentially be described as a "pro-inflammatory state".[34,35] Sleep apnoea, often seen in PCOS, is also seen as a "pro-inflammatory state".[36] Other chronic conditions seen in PCOS – metabolic syndrome, high blood pressure and diabetes – are also pro-inflammatory states.

Why has chronic dis-ease and inflammation become such an epidemic?[37,38] One theory is called the 'nutrition transition', or the switch from a vegetable and fruit-based food plan to one that is high in meat, sugar, saturated fats and salt.[39,40,41] Interestingly, an improved food plan, tobacco cessation and increased physical activity may prevent up to 80% of cases of coronary artery dis-ease and 90% of diabetes.[42] Other reasons cited for the increase in chronic dis-ease, and which increase free radical damage, include tobacco use, increased stress, environmental toxins and a lack of exercise. The increase in obesity – tied to all the other factors, of course, tends to be the single most common factor in chronic dis-ease.[43]

The last century has seen the rise of chronic dis-eases, known as 'the diseases of modern civilisation', some of which were never seen, or were exceedingly rare, before.[44,45,46,47] Ancient humans used to consume roughly the same amount of omega-6 and omega-3 fats. Studies indicate they ate about a 1:1 ratio.[48] Modern humans consume more than *15* times more omega-6 fats than omega-3 fats – a 15:1 ratio.[49] In some countries, people consume *20* times more omega-6 than omega-3! In those countries where the ratio of omega-6 to omega-3 is more than 4:1, there is a corresponding increase in chronic dis-ease.[50] Ancient humans died from trauma and infections, but they did NOT die from chronic dis-ease.

What does all of this have to do with PCOS? While we don't intricately understand all the mechanisms involved in the development of PCOS, oxidative stress and inflammation are two important drivers. As mentioned, conditions associated with PCOS, and PCOS itself, have been found to be connected to high levels of oxidative stress and the resulting inflammation.

Now, what can you *do* about it? One of the most important things you can do is adopt an anti-inflammatory food plan. Before we get into the types of foods that are anti-inflammatory, a word about omega-6 and omega-3 essential fatty acids is needed.

Essential fatty acids (EFAs) are a type of fatty acid that can't be made by your body and must be obtained from the foods you eat. If these fats are not in your food plan, they are not in your body.

Most important for their effects on inflammation are the omega-3, omega-6 and omega-9 fats. (The main source of omega-9 fats, an anti-inflammatory fat, is olive oil).

Omega-3 fats are used by the body to make substances that are *anti*-inflammatory (they reduce inflammation) while omega-6 fats tend to be funnelled into substances that are *pro*-inflammatory (they increase inflammation). The critical issue lies in the *ratio* of omega-6 and omega-3 fatty acids we ingest and absorb. Omega-6 fats are very readily found in foods – most vegetable oils, for example. Omega-6 fats are also found in high amounts in meat – particularly red meat from cows raised eating non-grass foods. The omega-3 fats, on the other hand are found mainly in fish. The tendency over the last century has been for increasing amounts of omega-6 fats relative to omega-3 fats in our food plan. It is this skewed ratio that is so very important, and tips the balance towards one of inflammation.

An anti-inflammatory food plan increases the amount of omega-3 fats, often by supplementing with fish oils. Olive oil is also included as the omega-9 fats in this oil have anti-inflammatory properties. Other anti-inflammatory foods include fruits, berries and vegetables (especially the leafy green variety), nuts, brown rice, lean (organic, free-range) poultry, wild-caught fish and seafood, soy foods such as tempeh, legumes such as lentils and beans, green tea, fruit and vegetable juices and a lot of pure water. Many herbs and spices are anti-inflammatory as well. You can use them in your cooking to add flavour and variety. These herbs and spices include curcumin, ginger, paprika, dill, mint, thyme, marjoram, oregano, basil, rosemary, parsley, celery, onions and garlic. Organic food is highly recommended. You can grow your own vegetables – this not only makes them affordable and guarantees better quality, but tending to your garden can be therapeutic as well. Simple, whole foods – as pesticide and toxin free as you can find – will not only reduce your inflammation and help you lose weight, the process of cooking the food also gives you control over what you eat and how you eat it.

Although we live in a vastly different world to the world of the past, we can improve many areas important in our health. It is a simple idea, yet not always so simple to incorporate into our lives. The fact is, eating more like your grandparents did can be a big boost to your health and vitality. Improving your anti-inflammatory lifestyle and decreasing your inflammation and oxidative stress will improve your PCOS, and so much more.

Can't get enough?

Go to *www.ConquerYourPCOSNaturally.com/ BonusReports* to grab your FREE bonuses.

As an additional bonus, you'll also receive Dr Rebecca's *'Conquer Your PCOS'* monthly newsletter for FREE. You'll discover even more PCOS advice, easy-to-apply practical tips, PCOS-friendly recipes, and become a *'Conquer Your PCOS'* VIP.

Act now and join us and the 'Conquer Your PCOS' community!

Also, follow Dr Rebecca at:

www.Facebook.com/ConquerYourPCOS
and
http://Twitter.com/ConquerPCOS

Chapter Eight

Toxicity Warning!

Learn why plastic water bottles and your favourite perfume could be contributing to your wayward hormones, infertility and even directly to your PCOS

> *"The future will depend on our wisdom not to replace one poison with another."*
>
> National Pediculosis Association®, Inc.

Toxicity is the ability of a chemical substance, drug or poison to produce harmful effects on a living organism, including you.

Toxicity can be:

- Acute, through an intense single short-term exposure.
- Chronic, through repeated or continuous exposure over a long period of time.
- Sub-chronic, through repetitive or continuous exposure over a period of more than 12 months.

As we create more pollution in our world, introduce toxins into our food and our drink, our personal and cleaning products, and create toxic input into our brains from faulty spinal movement, our toxic load increases.

In the US, tonnes of toxic industrial wastes, including

the likes of heavy metals, are being mixed with liquid agricultural fertilisers and being dispersed across American farmlands.[1]

An FDA investigation in 2004 found mercury residue in all of the mercury cell chlor-alkali products including caustic soda, chlorine, potassium hydroxide and hydrochloric acid. Mercury is recognised as a neurotoxic heavy metal.[2] This means is it toxic to the nervous system. Such is the impact of this substance that the American Academy of Pediatrics has recommended minimising any form of mercury exposure, noting this advice is essential for optimal child health and nervous system development.[3] Another study showed mercury can cross the placental barrier, and could be seen in the growing foetus.

Gender benders

To understand how toxicity influences our hormones, you may need to refer back to how your hormones and cell receptors work in Chapter 3 'Restore Your Hormonal Balance – Discover what your hormones do, and the secrets to balancing them once more.'

There are now man-made substances in the environment that can mimic the actions of your own hormones; these fake hormones are often referred to as 'xenohormones', or endocrine disruptors.

Gender benders can have both detrimental effects on your health, and can cause malformations in the reproductive systems of your babies.

Endocrine disruptors do just that. They upset your delicate hormonal balance. Similar in structure to hormones, they bind with the cell receptors. In this way, they can alter your hormonal balance, block your body's normal responses, increase hormonal activity (as xenoestrogens do), and alter the interaction between the hormones and their carrier proteins. For example, pyrethyroid insecticides can displace testosterone from its carrier proteins in the body.[4]

Some of the most important endocrine disruptors are:

- Pesticides/fungicides
- Lead
- Dioxin
- Dichloridiphenyl Trichloroethane (DDT)
- Polychlorinated biphenyl (PCB)
- Formaldehyde
- Solvents.

From damage to ovarian function, ovarian cysts, PCOS, immune disorders, depression and anxiety to infertility, cancer and endometriosis, these endocrine disruptors can cause, or contribute to, many disorders.

To better understand xenohormones, let's take a closer look at some of the most commonly found endocrine disruptors.

Persistent organic pollutants (POPs)

Persistent Organic Pollutants (POPs) can be:

- Industrial chemicals
- Pesticides
- Unwanted wastes.

POPs are products and by-products of industrial processes. POPs are released into the environment through air and water, travelling on wind and water currents.

POPs are toxic. They can accumulate in your body and your fat cells. They are difficult to break down, and remain in our bodies and our environment for a long time. Once released into the environment, they detrimentally affect our health, and the health of our planet.

Exposure to POPs

Being exposed to a POP is significant. Our modern environment and lifestyle means we are exposed to a concoction of many POPs, combined with other toxins, over a long period of time. Really, not at all good for us.

How do you become exposed to POPs?

1. Through the food chain

POPs are stored in the fatty tissues of animals and humans. As one animal eats another, these toxins continue to accumulate. By the time these POPs reach the top of the food chain – us – the amount ingested is compounded, and we receive the highest dose. This is the same for other toxins, such as mercury.

2. At birth, and through the mother's body

As a woman accumulates toxins through her life, she may pass these on to her child during its development in the womb and through breast-feeding. One study found toxic chemicals in the bodies of pregnant women.[5]

3. Through global winds and currents

Some POPs have the ability to contaminate regions very far from their original source, as they can be transported across regions via air currents. For example, some POPs originating from warmer regions of the globe can travel to the colder polar regions. Once there, they condense, precipitate and reach the earth's surface again.

List of POPs

Often referred to as the 'dirty dozen', there are 12 POPs suspected of persisting in our environment.

List of 12 key POPs

CHEMICAL OR CLASS	NOTES
ALDRIN	Pesticide widely used on corn and cotton until 1970. EPA allowed its use for termites until manufacturer cancelled registration in 1987. Closely related to dieldrin.
CHLORDANE	Pesticide on agricultural crops, lawns, and gardens and a fumigant for termite control. All uses were banned in the United States in 1988 but still produced for export.
DDT	Pesticide still used for malaria control in the tropics. Banned for all but emergency uses in the United States in 1972.
DIELDRIN	Pesticide widely used on corn and cotton until 1970. EPA allowed its use for termites until manufacturer cancelled registration in 1987. A breakdown product of aldrin.
ENDRIN	Used as a pesticide to control insects, rodents, and birds. Not produced or sold for general use in the United States since 1986.
HEPTACHLOR	Insecticide in household and agricultural uses until 1988. Also a component and a breakdown product of chlordane.
HEXACHLOROBENZENE (HCB)	Pesticide and fungicide used on seeds, also an industrial byproduct. Not widely used in the United States since 1965.
MIREX	Insecticide and flame retardant not used or manufactured in the United States since 1978.
TOXAPHENE	Insecticide used primarily on cotton. Most uses in the U.S. were banned in 1982, and all uses in 1990.
PCBs	Polychlorinated biphenyls, widely used in electrical equipment and other uses. Manufacture of PCBs banned in the United States in 1977.
POLYCHLORINATED DIOXINS and POLYCHLORINATED FURANS	Two notorious classes of "unintentional" pollutants, byproducts of incineration and industrial processes. Regulated in the United States under air, water, food quality, occupational safety, waste, and other statutes.

Source: http://www.uspopswatch.org/global/dirty-dozen.htm

Adapted from the Public Heath Statements on certain chemicals by Agency for Toxic Substances and Disease Registry, a part of the US Department of Health and Human Services.

Xenoestrogens

Simply put, xenoestrogens are a family of chemicals that can enter the body and mimic the action of our natural hormone, oestrogen. One type of endocrine disruptor – known as a xenoestrogen – acts by attaching itself to the oestrogen receptors on our cells. There they can then mimic our own oestrogen. As a result, your body essentially has too much oestrogen, and oestrogenic effects may be exerted at incorrect times.

An early onset of puberty, uterine fibroids, endometriosis, PMS and PCOS are just some of the examples of the negative effects xenoestrogens can have on your reproductive system.

So, where are all are these chemicals found?

Xenoestrogens – the key sources

Xenoestrogens can be found in:

- Soft plastics, such as cling wraps and food containers. As a rule, the softer the plastic, the greater the presence of such chemicals.
- Once a plastic is heated, xenoestrogens are released. Think about the bottle you drink your water from, the cling wrap you use in the microwave, or the lid on your morning take-away coffee.
- Birth control pills, containing doses of synthetic oestrogens.
- Pesticides and herbicides, including those you normally use in your home.
- Commercially available deodorants, shampoos, soaps and cosmetics.
- Commercially grown meat products.

Hormone-sensitive organs, such as the breast, are highly susceptible to damage from xenoestrogens. Research shows that the natural oestrogen 17β-estradiol and xenoestrogenic substances like bisphenol A are able to induce neoplastic transformation – potentially cancerous changes – in human breast epithelial cells.[6] Xenoestrogens may also displace endogenous sex steroid hormones from SHBG binding sites and disrupt the androgen-to-oestrogen balance.[7] This androgen-oestrogen balance is a significant issue for many women with PCOS.

Our toxic diet

Infertility and premature ovarian decline can result from the toxicity in the food we eat and the liquid we drink. How can dietary toxicity wreak havoc on our reproductive system, and act as an 'ovarian damager'?

Excitotoxins – the silent enemy

You no doubt know that junk food is bad for you. But, have you thought about how this 'food' and drink can really affect your hormones?

Excitotoxins, also known as neurotoxicants, are chemical substances capable of causing damage, or even death, to your nerve cells. When we consume this junk, these excitotoxins stimulate such intense and rapid firing of our nerve endings that the cells can run out of chemical messengers. The nerve cells in the hypothalamus (our master hormone and reproductive regulator) are most sensitive to this phenomenon. Shockingly, these excitotoxins can even start damaging the brain cells in the hypothalamus of the baby growing in the mother's womb.

> *"Junk food means junk in our bodies, in our brains,*
> *in our babies, in our communities and in our environment!"*
>
> *Dr Rebecca Harwin, PCOS Expert, Author and Chiropractor*

Reproductive toxicity – the impact

As with any species, we depend on reproduction for our survival and growth. Agents that produce reproductive toxicity can have an effect on the differentiation, development and adult functioning of the reproductive system of an individual.[8] Such reproductive toxins can have a vast series of impacts, including those listed below:

- Foetal death
- Impaired fertility
- Congenital problems
- Altered growth
- Malformation of reproductive structures
- Delayed or early reproductive developmental stages.

Research shows strong evidence of a correlation between such endocrine disruptors, POPs and chemical substances, discussed above, with dis-eases such as PCOS. A recent study reported that women with PCOS may be more vulnerable to exposure to the chemical bisphenol A (BPA), which is commonly found in many plastic household items.[9] A known endocrine disruptor, BPA is found in increased levels in women with PCOS, and is linked with higher levels of 'male' hormones in such women. This study found that as BPA blood levels increased, the concentrations of testosterone also increased in women with PCOS.

The following toxic substances can have a major impact on the reproductive systems at various stages of growth:

- Persistent organic pollutants (POPs), such as dioxins, PCBs, DDT.
- Heavy metals such as mercury, lead, manganese, arsenic and cadmium.
- Organic solvents such as toluene, benzene, xylene, acetone, vinyl chloride, trichloroethylene, phenols.
- Hormonally-active agents like plasticisers.
- Pesticides of such categories as carbamate and organophosphate.

What can you do to detoxify yourself and your environment?

Healthy nutritional choices and supplements, along with some key lifestyle changes can help you combat today's toxic onslaught.

Environmental pollution, food and drink toxicity, personal and cleaning products all create toxicity that needs to be minimised – if not eliminate – for your general health as well as your reproductive health.

We also create toxic input into our brains by faulty spinal movement, and by toxic thinking.

Eleven ways to fight the toxic effect:

1. Whenever possible, eat only certified organic fruits, vegetables, meats and gluten-free grains. Where appropriate, wash the raw produce before you cook or eat it.

2. Focus on consuming real foods. Most packaged and processed foods are not only not health-promoting, they also place additional stress on your body and use up valuable nutrients you need for health in the removal of their toxins.

3. Use only natural personal hygiene and cleaning products. Look out for these chemicals in the personal care products and cosmetics you use, and avoid them: benzophenone-3, homosalate, 4-methyl-benzylidene camphor (4-MBC), octyl-methoxycinnamate and octyl-dimethyl-PABA. Look for great companies that focus on ethical ingredients.

4. Eat foods high in fibre and cruciferous vegetables like broccoli, sprouts and cauliflower. These provide you with health promoting nutrients. They also help combat the impact of xenoestrogens, and assist in detoxifying your body.

5. Choose chlorine-free and unbleached paper products.

6. Avoid using plastic containers for heating or storing products. Avoid using plastic bottles for storing drinking water. Use glass containers instead.

7. Avoid inhaling noxious gases from copiers, printers, carpets, fibre boards, cars, perfumes, household sprays and gas pumps.

8. Use condoms without spermicides for birth control.

9. Stay away from perfumes, nail paints and nail polish removers.

10. Be wary of medications, limit alcohol, avoid drugs and stop smoking.

11. See your Chiropractor regularly to ensure the neurological input to your brain is not toxic (nociception).

Seven ways to protect your environment:

1. Become informed. Ask for information. There is power in knowledge.

2. Ask for non-toxic products at your grocery store. Find companies that specialise in health-promoting products.

3. Read packaging… or just avoid packaged foods.

4. Use only biodegradable, toxin-free detergents, personal care and cleaning products, and cosmetics.

5. Use items like bicarb of soda and vinegar as cleaning agents.

6. Support movements that advocate phasing out harmful chemicals in the environment.

7. Spread information and awareness among your loved ones.

Can't get enough?

Go to *www.ConquerYourPCOSNaturally.com/BonusReports* to grab your FREE bonuses.

As an additional bonus, you'll also receive Dr Rebecca's *'Conquer Your PCOS'* monthly newsletter for FREE. You'll discover even more PCOS advice, easy-to-apply practical tips, PCOS-friendly recipes, and become a *'Conquer Your PCOS'* VIP.

Act now and join us and the 'Conquer Your PCOS' community!

Also, follow Dr Rebecca at:

www.Facebook.com/ConquerYourPCOS
and
http://Twitter.com/ConquerPCOS

Chapter Nine

Your Thyroid

*How to boost your metabolism,
have abundant energy and lose weight*

The thyroid gland – the metabolic engine of your body

"I feel tired. It's so hard to get motivated to exercise, not to mention my muscles hurt so much. I just can't lose weight. I feel depressed, my skin really sucks, and if I could just remember..."

Does any of this sound familiar? These symptoms could actually be a sign of something more challenging.

> *A little goes a long way.*
>
> *A small amount of hormone makes a big difference.*
>
> *Did you know your thyroid only makes approximately one teaspoon of thyroid hormone each year?*
>
> *Amazingly, this tiny amount is sufficient to affect each and every cell in your body.*

What is your thyroid?

Your thyroid is a small gland that sits at the base of your neck, just in front of your windpipe and below your voice box. It's shaped like a butterfly – appropriately 'girly' – as thyroid problems affect five to eight times more women than men.[1]

Usually less than an ounce in weight, your thyroid is made up of two lobes, right and left. The functions of your thyroid gland are controlled by the pituitary gland, which is, in turn, controlled by your hypothalamus (both located in your brain).

The thyroid gland has one of the richest blood supplies in our body. A giant volume of four to five litres (8.5 to 10.5 pints) of blood flows through this teensy little gland every hour!

Body Structures & Functions, by Ann Senisi Scott, Elizabeth Fong, Cengage Learning, 2009, p207.

What does the thyroid gland do?

Although small in size, you should not underestimate the importance of this gland. Your thyroid is vital for maintaining your health and keeping the 'spark' in your life. This tiny gland releases powerful hormones, which help in controlling and releasing energy for all of your metabolic processes.

To cut a long story short, your thyroid gland is the metabolic engine of your body. It ubiquitously affects every cell in your body. Your thyroid:

- Can modify how your genes are expressed
- Regulates your metabolism by regulating the use of glucose and oxygen for the production of heat and energy
- Regulates the speed of your enzymes
- Regulates bone mass by affecting calcium metabolism
- Regulates cholesterol and fat metabolism
- Is involved in the regulation of your reproductive functions.

How does this tiny gland do such a mammoth task?

When it comes to the thyroid, the immense strength of this gland lies in the potent hormones it releases in your blood. The three hormones of the thyroid gland are:

- Thyroxin
- Tri-iodothyronine
- Calcitonin.

The secretions of these hormones are regulated by thyroid stimulating hormone or TSH, secreted by the pituitary gland. The hypothalamus in turn regulates the release of TSH from the pituitary by releasing the TSH-releasing hormone (TRH). This communication between your hypothalamus, pituitary gland and thyroid gland is called your Hypothalamic-Pituitary-Thyroid Axis (or HPT). Development of the HPT is crucial for reproduction and overall development in men as well as women.[2]

When the levels of your thyroid hormones drop, your hypothalamus tells the pituitary gland to produce more TSH. The opposite occurs when your thyroid hormone levels get too high. This system, known as a 'negative feedback' system, is used by most of our body's endocrine glands for ensuring balance – or homeostasis.

Why should you know more about this gland?

The thyroid is an extremely important gland due not only to its impact on your overall health, but also as it affects your menstruation, ovulation and fertility. PCOS and hypothyroidism have also been linked.[3,4]

According to Evanthia Diamanti-Kandarakis – co-author of *Insulin Resistance and Poly Cystic Ovarian Syndrome: Pathogenesis, Evaluation, and Treatment*, p325, "decreased SHBG and increased free testosterone levels and altered estradiol metabolism have been described in hypothyroid patients, whereas PCO has been detected in 36.5% of hypothyroid patients". The authors believe hypothyroidism may enhance the PCOS phenotype, meaning an underactive thyroid may change how your genes are expressed to those resembling a PCOS pattern.[5] For more detailed information about gene expression, see Chapter 2 'Is PCOS In Your Genes? – Learn how to control your genes to be healthy instead of sick'.

A condition called thyroid autoimmune dis-ease (whereby one's own body creates rogue anti-bodies that destroy the thyroid, leading to thyroid imbalance) is three times more common in women with PCOS than those without. It is also the most common autoimmune disorder in women and is a major reason behind unexplained infertility.[6]

Trying to conceive with a lousy thyroid can be difficult. Combine PCOS and suboptimal thyroid function and you have challenges in not only becoming pregnant, but maintaining a healthy pregnancy and safely delivering a healthy child. Excessive thyroid hormones i.e. hyperthyroidism can cause miscarriage and unexplained infertility.[7] Lowered production of thyroid hormones i.e. hypothyroidism can lead to irregular periods, infertility, anovulation, and a sluggish body. If you're feeling sluggish and slow, your eggs are feeling just the same way. In fact, the only thing speeding up in hypothyroidism is the ageing process.

The mindboggling functions of T3 and T4

Nurture growth: Thyroid hormones along with growth hormones are critical for normal growth and bone development.[8] They are also very important for the normal development of the nervous system. A deficiency of thyroid hormones during pregnancy and in the early years of life, can lead to mental retardation, intelligence deficits and seizures.[9] Poor supply of thyroid hormones in early life leads to stunted growth; a condition known as the 'thyroid dwarf' or cretinism.

Accelerate metabolism: Thyroid hormones have 'calorigenic' action. Meaning, they accelerate oxygen and energy consumption in all the active tissues of the body and pump-up the Basal Metabolic Rate (BMR). The higher the BMR, the higher the rate of calories burnt. Thyroid hormones regulate the use of glucose, fats and proteins in our body for energy production.[10] Lower levels of thyroid hormone lead to lower energy levels, and so lethargy and sluggishness.

Conversely, too much thyroid hormone is also a cause for concern. Abnormally high levels of thyroid hormones will make you jumpy, irritable, and fatigued and you may experience light or absent periods, palpitations and increased bowel movements.

Thyroid hormone balance is needed to maintain body weight. Excessive thyroid hormone can lead to abnormal weight loss, and muscle mass loss. On the other hand, a deficiency can result in abnormal weight gain. Some studies suggest that an increase in the levels of TSH can cause central obesity that actually mimics the obesity of PCOS.[11] Hence, normalising the function of your thyroid hormones is the first step towards achieving adequate weight loss.

> ## Dirty nails?
>
> *Hyperthyroidism also causes a condition called 'Plummer's nails'. Abnormally high levels of thyroid hormones lead to separation of the front end of the nails. Dirt lodges deep into these raised spaces and is often difficult to clean; giving you perpetually dirty looking nails.*
>
> *Some thyroid conditions can also give you yellow green discoloration of the nails.*
>
> Thyroid Disorders with Cutaneous Manifestations, *by Warren Heymann, Springer, 2008, p171.*

'Gut' feeling: Thyroid hormones impact on our digestive system. They control the rate at which food moves through our intestines, and the rate of the absorption of essential nutrients from the digested food.[12] Increased appetite and excessive bowel movements can occur in hyperthyroidism. Hypothyroidism on the other hand may lead to poor or no appetite, and constipation.

Aesthetic effects: Thyroid hormones are responsible for the health of our skin, hair and nails. They promote production of oil and normal sweat. The growth and texture of our hair and nails is also dependent on thyroid hormones. It is not surprising that abnormal thyroid levels often present with abnormalities of skin, hair and nails. Hyperthyroidism may cause flushing of skin, warm and moist skin, due to hyperactive sweat and oil glands. It also affects the hair and nails, leading to hair loss, sparse, fine hair and brittle nails.[13]

Hypothyroidism may cause loss of the outer third of your eyebrows, hair loss, brittle or thin nails and dry skin.

Reproductive connection: Your thyroid hormones affect your reproductive system. Some of their major effects are on:

- Oestrogen and progesterone metabolism
- Female sexual maturation
- Regulation of the menstrual cycle
- Maintenance of ovulation and fertility
- Ability to reach a full-term pregnancy
- Appropriate production of follicle stimulating hormone (FSH).

Thyroid hormones play an astounding role in maintaining the hormonal balance in women. T3 stimulates the production of Sex Hormone Binding Globulin (SHBG), which is important for clearing circulating male hormones like testosterone from our blood.[14] Many women with PCOS have low levels of SHBG and high levels of free testosterone.

Calcitonin: Living up to its name, this hormone helps in maintaining the balance of calcium in our body. It prevents abnormal loss of calcium from our bones.[15]

T3 rules!

Tri-iodothyronine (T3) is three to eight times more potent than T4-thyronine. Its actions are much more rapid than T4. Although your thyroid makes four-fifths more T4 than T3, T3 has a far stronger effect on your body. Your thyroid makes 80% T4 and just 20% T3. Most of the T3 needed by the body is produced by converting T4 to T3.

T4 has four iodine molecules and T3 has three. Some of your T3 is made by your thyroid, but most is converted from T4 in your body. This conversion happens mainly in your liver and kidneys but, due to the importance of T3 to your body, conversion can occur in virtually every cell.

Cleaving the fourth iodine molecule on T4 converts it into the more powerful T3 hormone. Eighty per cent of T3 required by the body is produced by this mechanism. T4 is important, however. It serves as a storehouse for the supply of T3 as and when required.[16]

The tell-tale signs of thyroid disorders

People with thyroid disorders can have an overactive thyroid (hyperthyroidism) or an underactive thyroid (hypothyroidism).

Overactive thyroid: *Hyper*thyroidism is not as common as *hypo*thyroidism. It is five to 10 times more common in women than men. Some of the signs of hyper-thyroidism[17] are:

- Emotional liability, irritability
- Disturbed sleep
- Heat intolerance
- Weight loss
- Sweating
- Palpitations
- Bulging of the eyes
- Swelling over the thyroid
- Excessive thirst and appetite.

Women with PCOS are more likely to experience hypothyroidism. The common tell-tale signs of hypothyroidism[18,19] are:

Fatigue, lethargy	Dry skin and hair
Muscle weakness, pain & cramps	Hair loss from scalp and eyebrows
Cold intolerance, cold hands/feet	Slowed heartbeat / pulse
Goiter (swelling over the thyroid)	Hoarse voice
Weight gain	Dizziness or vertigo
Frequent infections	Poor memory, poor concentration
Depression	Chronic constipation
Puffiness around the eyes	Irritability
Menstrual irregularities and infertility	Throat pain, or a tender feeling
High cholesterol	Slow reflexes
'Brain fog' and indecisiveness	Fluid retention

Subclinical hypothyroidism: The current reference range used medically to indicate an under-performing thyroid is not what best evidence suggests. In Australia, the 'ideal range' for TSH is listed as between 0.5–4IU/L. Research shows a more accurate range would be between 1 to 2–2.5IU/L.[20] If you fall above 2.5IU/L, you are more likely to develop clinical hypothyroidism (as measured at above 4IU/L) in the future[21,22], and you may already be suffering from hypothyroid symptoms. I believe we should be seeing levels of TSH above 2–2.5IU/L as evidence of suboptimal thyroid status. Two to 3% of women suffer from this condition. Also, the risk increases with age.[23]

Like PCOS, subclinical hypothyroidism causes various pregnancy complications and increases the risk of preterm deliveries by almost two-fold.[24,25] Hodes noted an increased miscarriage risk in women with untreated hypothyroidism as far back as 1953. Also, this condition can lead to early pregnancy loss.[26]

Does hypothyroidism cause PCOS?

The 'cysts' in poly 'cystic' ovary syndrome are in fact immature follicles. Hypothyroidism causes decreased follicle stimulating hormone (FSH) levels. Low FSH causes immature follicles and unreleased eggs. Women with PCOS often have low absolute or relative FSH levels.

Thyroid autoimmune dis-ease (TAI)

Our immune system makes anti-bodies to destroy invaders. This is very important for our survival. Whether due to a food intolerance, toxin overload, or reasons we do not yet truly understand, sometimes a body may make anti-bodies against its own cells – known as auto-antibodies. Having thyroid auto-antibodies means having antibodies that destroy your very own thyroid gland. Longer term, this causes a deficiency of thyroid hormones, creating a hypothyroid state.

Many researchers have linked TAI to food allergies. A significant number of people with TAI have gluten intolerance.[27] Urticarial rash (an allergic skin condition) is common in people with TAI.[28]

Why harp over antibodies?

TAI is not an uncommon finding in women with PCOS. Conception is often more challenging when one has hypothyroidism and PCOS; having TAI poses further challenges. Even if you manage to become pregnant, thyroid auto-antibodies can cause recurrent miscarriages.[29]

Taking care of your thyroid

1.   Get yourself tested

The first step in thyroid care is to get your thyroid function tested. The battery of blood tests you need taken include – TSH, T4, T3, rT3 (reverse T3) and thyroid antibodies. There are functional pathology centres specialising in this kind of testing. Your health care professional can refer you.

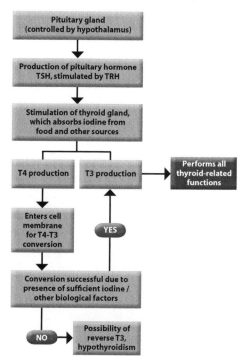

What is reverse T3 (rT3)?

When T4 is converted to the active T3, it loses one specific iodine molecule. If the iodine molecule T4 loses is the wrong one, you still get T3. But there is a hitch... this form of T3 is inactive. Reverse T3 in an inactive form of T3. If reverse T3 is not tested, you can test 'within normal limits' for your thyroid hormones and still suffer from hypothyroidism.

The mechanism of rT3

Remember, T3 is the worker that 'gets the job done'. rT3, on the other hand, is like a lazy, inactive sibling. Both T3 and rT3 can attach to the same receptors. Essentially, inactive rT3 can block the doorway and stop the worker, T3, from entering and getting the job done. Dr Wilson suggests that increased conversion of T4 to rT3 instead of the active T3 (Wilson's Syndrome), can occur due to significant physical and mental stress[30], calorie restriction or fasting, toxicity from prolonged and too much alcohol intake, or from heavy metals like mercury, lead and increased inflammation due to conditions like obesity.[31]

Are all these tests really that necessary?

Your TSH and T4 levels may fall 'within normal limits' on a standard medical blood test. You may be convinced – on past advice – that your thyroid is in good health. However, you may still be suffering from hypothyroidism. I see this in clinical practice.

Remember that T4 is not the most active thyroid hormone. It needs to lose one iodine molecule to become T3. Normally, this conversion is orchestrated by certain enzymes (5 deiodinase) along with dietary factors like tyrosine, iodine, selenium, zinc and omega-3. If this conversion is suboptimal, you will be a 'poor converter', with normal T4 yet deficient active T3. With the active thyroid hormone below normal levels, you are likely to suffer from subclinical hypothyroidism even with normal TSH and T4.[32]

Crash diets that starve you of calories may be one reason behind decreased active T3 production.[33] Such diets assault not just your thyroid, but almost every cell of your body. These diets create stress in your body, and push you further away from reaching your ideal weight.

More detailed thyroid information is included in the 'Conquering Your PCOS' 12-week home study course found at www.ConquerYourPCOSCourse.com

2.   Stock up on iodine

Iodine is critical to the health of your thyroid.

The thyroid is your body's main store of iodine. Apart from maintaining the thyroid functions, iodine plays a much bigger role in your body. Iodine is important for your immune function, cancer prevention, for the growth and development of your baby, both in your womb and during early infancy.

Guidelines issued by WHO and UNICEF recommend the following daily intakes of iodine to maintain optimal balance.[34]

- 0–7 years: 90μg (micrograms or millionths of a gram)
- 7–12 years: 120μg
- Older than 12 years/adult males and females: 150μg
- Pregnant and lactating women: 250μg.

As we discussed earlier, iodine deficiency in pregnancy can cause brain damage in your child.[35] An Australian study concluded that pregnant women and breastfeeding mothers in states such as NSW, Victoria, Tasmania and South Australia are likely to be iodine deficient.[36] Also, an estimated 31.5% of school-age children worldwide are iodine deficient.[37] This is an alarming statistic. Our next generation of children are at serious risk of the neuropsychological consequences of iodine deficiency!

The way we farm our food, and unfair pressure placed on farmers to produce food cheaply (would it not be more simple to pay farmers to tend and love our soils, and replace lost nutrients, than to later have the exorbitant costs associated with a needlessly suffering population?) has impacted our lands and given us substandard soil from which we can only reap substandard food. Such devastation of our farm soils, deforestation, our sub-par food plans, and exposure to toxins such as bromine, fluoride and chloride (which successfully compete with iodine for its receptor sites and 'toss it out of the game'), all contribute to iodine deficiency.

Getting iodine the right way!

Here is a simple test of common sense. If lack of iodine is responsible for the suboptimal functioning of your thyroid, do you think it is better to take a toxic drug to add synthetic thyroid hormone, or simply increase your dietary iodine intake?

Some of the best natural sources of iodine are:

- Seaweeds like dulse and kelp (pure and high quality) along with a wide assortment of sea foods.

> *Thyroid, iodine and breast cancer connection!*
>
> *Researchers believe there is a definite link between 'autoimmune thyroid disease', iodine consumption and the risk of breast cancer in women. The presence of autoimmune dis-ease increases the risk of breast cancer. A diet rich in iodine can prevent breast cancer. This explains the low rate of this deadly dis-ease in Japanese women, who eat plenty of seaweed and other iodine rich sea foods in their food plan.*
>
> The Thyroid, Iodine and Breast Cancer, *by Peter PA Smyth, Breast Cancer Research 2003, 5:235-23.*

- Natural sea salt is the best source of iodine in food (not refined salt with the addition of iodine).

3. More nutrients for better thyroid hormone function

- Proteins, especially those coming from fish like cold-water fish and lean animal proteins.

- Omega-3 fats such as those from high quality fish oil.

- Fruits and vegetables rich in antioxidant vitamins like vitamin A and C.

- Vitamin E from Swiss chard, mustard greens, sunflower seeds, almonds etc.

- Zinc from oysters, crabs, organic/grass-fed lean beef, sesame seeds and pumpkin seeds.

- Selenium from fish like cod, halibut, snapper and shrimp and from vegetarian sources like oats, sunflower seeds and brown rice etc.

- Tyrosine is an amino acid from chicken, turkey, fish, almonds, avocado, lima beans, pumpkin and sesame seeds.

- Magnesium from nuts, oranges, a little dark chocolate, passionfruit.

See your bonus special report 'What If The Foods Already In Your Cupboard Could Help You Conquer Your PCOS?' at *www. ConquerYourPCOSNaturally.com/BonusReports*

Boost your essential nutrients from foods in their most natural form. Organically grown food is better – it's more nutritious and less toxic. Supplement with high quality supplements where needed.

4. Watering your thyroid

Water is yet another critical factor when it comes to thyroid health. Normal drinking tap water is often fortified with fluoride and chloride. Both these chemicals are 'halogens' i.e. they belong to the same family of elements as iodine. They compete with iodine in our body. This can disrupt our thyroid function.

Drinking at least eight cups of pure filtered water a day is essential for optimum thyroid function.[38]

5. Supplements to help your thyroid to thrive

Often we need supplemental help to boost our thyroid function. Our soils lack important nutrients, we ingest detrimental anti-nutrients like bromine, and modern day stress and inflammation mean our nutrients, even when we receive them, are being diverted from our thyroid for use in other areas of our health. Remember, toxicity and/or deficiency is responsible for illness. This is also true for your thyroid.

Can't get enough?

Go to *www.ConquerYourPCOSNaturally.com/ BonusReports* to grab your FREE bonuses.

As an additional bonus, you'll also receive Dr Rebecca's *'Conquer Your PCOS'* monthly newsletter for FREE. You'll discover even more PCOS advice, easy-to-apply practical tips, PCOS-friendly recipes, and become a *'Conquer Your PCOS'* VIP.

Act now and join us and the 'Conquer Your PCOS' community!

Also, follow Dr Rebecca at:

www.Facebook.com/ConquerYourPCOS
and
http://Twitter.com/ConquerPCOS

Chapter Ten

Your Thoughts

You can think your way to improved health,
weight loss and a higher self-esteem

Women with PCOS are more likely to suffer from depression, anxiety and low self-esteem. We will discuss this later in this chapter. First, I wish to start by impressing upon you the importance of what and how you think. Hundreds of years ago, it was accepted that our mind and our body were inseparable. Each one affects and effects the other. Sadly, somewhere along the way, we lost our focus on the importance of mental, emotional and spiritual health. We somehow detached our physical self from these other selves. This was, and is, a grave error.

The mind and body connection – how we can begin to heal ourselves

There is a way of thinking that is both ancient and new. This way focuses on the interactions between the mind and the body, and takes into account the physical, emotional, mental, social, behavioural and spiritual sides of us, and how these affect our health. Historically, healers and medicine men were also the spiritual guides and mentors.[1] Traditional Chinese Medicine (TCM) has always considered the whole person and has approached healing by recognising that the mind, body and spirit affect each other in many ways.[2]

More recently, many healers and scientists have begun to look at the mind-body connection again, through the lens of biochemistry, biology, neurology and physiology. One of the first 'hints' that our thoughts can affect our bodies was through the work of Candace Pert. In the early 1980s, her research showed our immune system is affected by our emotions.[3] For example, when you are stressed, depressed or anxious, you tend to 'get sick' more often. There are now constant discoveries on the interrelationships between the way we think, and the impacts this has on our physical, mental, emotional, spiritual and social health. Studies on women having trouble becoming pregnant have shown those women who participated in the counselling, therapy or a support group had a significant increase in their fertility rates.[4]

There has also recently been a 'revolution' in the way many scientists look at our genes. This revolution proves, once again, we are designed to be *well*, not sick. Our genes are altered by what and how we eat – or don't eat, our movement, or lack thereof, our internal and external environment and by the way we think and feel.[5,6] This is the expanding field of epigenetics. Flick back to Chapter 2 'Is PCOS In Your Genes? – Learn how to control your genes to be healthy instead of sick' for a more detailed refresher on epigenetics. How you feel, what you think, your beliefs, and the stress you live under, all deeply affect your genetic expression.[7] Epigenetic changes are not mutations, the DNA sequence is not changed. Epigenetic changes *are reversible* – however, they can be passed down to your children. These changes occur from the ways that we respond to our environment,[8,9] including emotionally. The important thing to remember is that you *can* control aspects of your environment. You can change how you respond to events. This means *you* have control over the way your brain and body responds.

Let's look at some examples of how food affects our genetic

expression.[10,11,12] We can then expand on how your thoughts affect this. Folate, a B vitamin, represents one of the most well understood mechanisms. Folate is involved in a number of biochemical reactions that can control the effects of various gene products. Folate deficiency increases the risk of some cancers, heart dis-ease, neurological disorders and birth defects.[13] If you eat a diet rich in folate, or supplement with folate, these risks are decreased because the genes at the core of these disorders are suppressed.[14] Overeating or obesity can also affect how genes are expressed, often starting when an individual is very young – or even still in the womb.[15,16,17]

Stress and behaviour can also affect how our genes are expressed.[18,19,20,21,22] What's more, how we behave, think and feel and, of course, our food plan can *also* affect a child while a woman is pregnant. These *in utero* changes can affect the child through to adulthood, and throughout their entire life. They may even be passed down to *their* children![23,24] Do you see how important this is? Your lifestyle, and your thoughts, may affect your grandchildren and beyond.

So, what can be done about this? How can we control the way our genes are expressed? The short answer is by our food, movement, meditation, relaxation, self-belief, positive thinking, changing any misguided beliefs and improving our environment. For example, a recent study was conducted on men with prostate cancer.[25] After a three-month period – which included retreats, meditation, stress reduction, relaxation, a whole food diet that was low fat, low in refined carbohydrates and high in fruits, vegetables, unrefined grains, legumes plus a weekly support group – it was shown that *the DNA from blood cells had changed!* In many ways, these were not the same men who had started the study. They had a healthier immune system, felt stronger, felt happier *and* showed clinical improvements. These same types of improvements can be seen in PCOS as well. By following a similar food and stress reduction plan to the one mentioned in the prostate study, that is by increasing fibre, decreasing refined carbohydrates, decreasing unhealthy fats and increasing healthy fats such as omega-3 and omega-9 fatty acids, and decreasing stress, women with PCOS not only lost weight, but also decreased the amounts of testosterone[26], reduced their risk of diabetes[27] and heart dis-ease.[28] I hope you are learning that the lifestyle, including your thinking, needed to conquer your PCOS is also the lifestyle needed for optimal health and vital well-being. This is also the lifestyle required for any human to be well.

I need to clarify one thing with regard to your thoughts. This is not a 'just think positive thoughts and it'll be okay' approach. It is not easy to change your beliefs, your thoughts and your responses. It is not always easy, but it *is* entirely possible and absolutely necessary if you are to be well. Change takes time to implement, especially when you are looking to change thought habits and emotions. Healing is a process, not an event. Be patient with yourself. You need to be consistent... the important thing to remember is that *you* are in control and *you* decide. And *you,* the people around you, and your future children will be the ones that benefit. One very helpful approach is to find others in the same position – call it a support group, or a circle of supportive friends. Having people around who understand and support you is very important in the process of change. A counsellor can offer invaluable assistance in this process, and give you the tools needed to succeed.

Bruce Lipton, cell biologist, researcher and writer, has written extensively on how to achieve some of these goals, how to teach yourself and, perhaps more importantly, how to allow yourself to heal by not only changing the foods you eat and the environment in which you live, but also by teaching yourself how to use conscious belief to change your perceptions of your mental, emotional and physical health.[29,30] *The Biology of Belief* and *Spontaneous*

Evolution: Our Positive Future (and a Way to Get There From Here) are two books I strongly recommended as you continue on this journey. They provide the understanding to allow you to take control and a plan to put this control into action. Another helpful reference is Dawson Church's *The Genie in Your Genes – Epigenetic Medicine and the New Biology of Intention.*[31]

What you believe will determine your success

What you think matters... or, more correctly, what you *believe* matters. What you believe determines what you think and how you behave. Most people think their thoughts are their own. But is that entirely true?

Most of what you believe, what forms your 'habits', does not arise from your conscious thinking brain – the brain you are aware of. Most comes from your subconscious brain. The kicker is, most of the knowledge in your subconscious brain was 'downloaded' when you were young. The things you observed/heard/ experienced when you were very young have shaped your view of yourself and your world today.

When you are very young, you spend more time using brain waves different to those you predominantly use as an adult. Plus, the part of your brain that is involved in learning is constantly 'on'. If this was not the case, you could not have learned the substantial amount of knowledge you needed to learn. At this time, you also do not use the 'filters' we develop as we age – you accept what you see/hear/experience to be true. As an adult, if you are told you are an idiot, you have filters that can rationalise this information. You can (providing you have not been conditioned to think this to be true) filter that statement and know it is incorrect. When you are an impressionable child, however, this filter isn't switched on. Can you imagine the damage this can do?

Now back to you, today. Most of your habits – your thoughts – come from the information you downloaded as a child. Most of what you downloaded was from the input of other people. So, the programming in your subconscious brain – the part of your brain that forms your habits and your beliefs, the part that really runs your life – is *not* of your making.

Why is this relevant to you and PCOS?

You may make a choice consciously, say, to lose weight. You will, invariably, find you need to rely on 'willpower' – the conscious brain's ability to override your subconscious brain for a time. But, if your subconscious brain has different views to your conscious brain, you will not 'win' long-term. You have, I'm sure, heard of self-sabotage. These are harsh words, for your brain reverting to what it 'knows' to be true.

Unless you realise that most of the programs running you are not those you consciously downloaded, but those learned from the input of other people, you may find it very difficult to succeed. The subconscious brain is *so* much bigger, *so* much more powerful, than your conscious brain!

If you want to make real change in your life, you need to stop blaming yourself. You need to stop believing you are weak, that you don't have the willpower to succeed. Even that you don't deserve to succeed. You need to work to change your subconscious programming. This is the way to make real change.

What you think does matter, but it's what you believe that determines what you think and so how you act.

Remember, thoughts – both positive and negative – affect your state of mind, your state of being *and* your state of health. There will be times when you feel more negatively. Everyone gets angry, scared, frustrated or sad at times. The key is to recognise it, acknowledge it, take steps to move forward and then let it go. Then, replace it with joy, belief, love, affirmation, and the recognition that the next time, it will be easier and the next time, you will be healthier.

I also need to address mental health.

Depressed, anxious, fearful, stressed... do any, or all, of these describe the way you feel? Are you scared, lonely, shy, shamed, do you feel worthless or unattractive? Have you lost all interest in the things you used to do? Is it difficult to wake up or go to sleep? Have you even thought about death or dying?

People may say 'I'm depressed' when they are having a tough day, when what they mean is 'I'm fed up', 'today sucks', 'I feel grumpy'. This is not clinical depression. But when that depressed feeling lasts longer and causes emotional, physical and behavioural changes, it is time to seek help. Disturbances in sleep and appetite, headache, tummy ache, loss of energy, loss of interest in activities that once were enjoyed, crying without reason, feeling hopeless, guilty, worthless, irritable, empty or even suicidal, may indicate clinical depression. Clinical depression interferes with activities of daily living.[32] There may have been a major change or life stress. This stress may be obvious, such as divorce, changing a job, being in an accident, going through a major disaster, or losing a family member or friend. However, depression is not always so clear cut. It is important to realise that depression is *not* just temporary sadness. Clinical depression can last your entire life, with some good days and more bad days, and can affect everything you do. Major depression is disabling and can keep you from functioning at a job, or with family and friends.

So what causes depression? We don't understand that completely – there are chemical changes in the brain that are associated with depression.[33,34,35,36,37] These are associated with changes in a number of substances that transmit messages to different nerve cells in the brain, the neurotransmitters.[38,39,40] These neurotransmitters include substances like serotonin, GABA, epinephrine and norepinephrine. People with depression have also been found to have changes in the size of certain parts of their brain. Recent research is looking to chronic stress as a likely cause of depression. If someone in your family has had depression, you are more likely to have depression also.[41] Women are more likely than men to suffer from depression.[42,43] Also, your environment – including the people you live with, the work you do and the area you live in can all affect the risk of depression. If you live in an unhealthy or abusive relationship, or if you live on the edge financially, this increases your risk of depression.[44]

Depression – and anxiety – can be associated with any major medical condition, including PCOS.[45,46,47,48] Depression often occurs along with anxiety.[49] Anxiety indicates an over-reaction and concern or worry about everyday situations, or worrying about an unlikely situation. In anxiety, the reaction to a situation appears to others to be excessive, and may be accompanied by physical symptoms such as fatigue, headaches, muscle aches or tension, a dry mouth and/or difficulty in swallowing, sleep problems, nausea or vomiting, trembling or twitching in the arms, legs or face, irritability or mood swings, sweating, a severe startle reflex and hot flashes.[50,51] Anxiety can be disabling. Both the depression and anxiety you may be feeling can be related to your condition – but, just as you can take a proactive stance to improve your physical health, you can take proactive steps to improve your mental health.

What can you do to address depression and anxiety?

Professor Irving Kirsch studied the effectiveness of anti-depressant medications in detail. He found antidepressants were as effective, but clinically not significantly different, to that of placebo (or 'sugar pills').[52]

So, what does help?

Counselling. Exercise. Community. Increasing those nutrients required for making our happy hormones, like B6, Zinc and omega-3.

Remember also, your physical, mental, emotional and spiritual health are intertwined, not separate.

Can't get enough?

Go to *www.ConquerYourPCOSNaturally.com/ BonusReports* to grab your FREE bonuses.

As an additional bonus, you'll also receive Dr Rebecca's *'Conquer Your PCOS'* monthly newsletter for FREE. You'll discover even more PCOS advice, easy-to-apply practical tips, PCOS-friendly recipes, and become a *'Conquer Your PCOS'* VIP.

Act now and join us and the 'Conquer Your PCOS' community!

Also, follow Dr Rebecca at:

www.Facebook.com/ConquerYourPCOS
and
http://Twitter.com/ConquerPCOS

Chapter Eleven

The Magic Of Movement

How to simply and easily incorporate movement into your life. Plus, I reveal the single training tip for quicker, easier fat loss and hormonal control

We were designed to move, to work for our food, to run from threats. But movement is much more than this. Movement is crucial to life. Somewhere along the way, as life sped up and we slowed down, we all but lost this most important nutrient. That's right; movement is a *critical nutrient* for our health. Movement affects how our brain functions, our organs work, our cells receive their critical communication and how our genes express themselves. Movement helps us maintain our balance, our homeostasis. Without it, we simply cannot lead a healthy, fulfilling, productive and happy life.

Correct movement is also crucial for you in conquering your PCOS.

Let's look at why...

- For all animals, including human beings, movement is critical to be well. This should be your *primary focus* to achieve a long, healthy, happy life.
- Exercise induces normal expression of the genome.[1] In other words, exercise lets your genes work as they are designed to.

- Lack of exercise can manifest in metabolic syndrome.[2] Important for everyone, not just a woman with PCOS, I'm sure you'd agree.
- Type 2 diabetes, coronary heart dis-ease, stroke, hypertension and many cancers could be prevented/ improved with exercise.
- Exercise improves your basal metabolic rate (BMR). Your BMR is the rate at which your body uses energy to maintain your vital functions, while at rest. The higher your BMR, the more energy you use. This translates into less energy being stored.
- Inactivity results in dyslipidemia (higher LDL and decreased HDL levels, higher triglycerides).
- Movement helps us use the nutrients we ingest.
- Exercise helps our bowels move correctly, and removes toxins.
- Movement creates our 'happy hormones' and helps normalise our stress levels.
- Exercise helps clear the head.
- Exercise encourages us to be rational, and can normalise mood swings.
- Movement is motivating.
- Exercise can quash cravings.
- Exercise helps us use insulin correctly.
- Inactivity results in glucose and insulin remaining in the blood longer after a meal, than in those who are active.
- Insulin Resistance increases after a few days of physical inactivity.[3]
- Exercise helps maintain an ideal weight.
- Exercise helps keep your bones strong.
- Exercise maintains the active muscle mass we need in order to function optimally.

- Inactivity reduces immune function.
- Exercise is anti-ageing.
- Movement decreases pain.

... It's incredibly important to talk about the affect correct movement has on your brain. As you know, your brain is the overseer, the coordinator, of the health and balance in all the cells and systems of your body.

So, what increases your brain function?

Physical activity and Chiropractic! Both of these focus on optimising your health and well-being, and improving your brain function. It is a much better focus for you, eliminating toxicity and deficiency to attain purity and sufficiency. This is not only the way to conquer your PCOS, it is also the way to achieve balance and restore true health.

Objectives of your movement program

Your efforts in regard to movement are critical. Apart from moving you towards true health, movement has so many benefits for you in conquering your PCOS. You will feel less stressed and have less cravings, moving will help to normalise your hormones, and moving will have you well on your way to creating a new you.

There are three parts to moving correctly: exercise, Chiropractic and correct posture.

Physical activity

Physical activity is so much more important than simply gaining the upper hand in weight loss, or in looking good.

For example, regular exercise significantly lowered the level of homocysteine – a toxic waste product linked to heart dis-ease – in the blood of young overweight women suffering from PCOS.[4]

The evidence base supporting the notion that moving well changes and improves your function is now almost endless.

Let's look at how exercise helps women gain control of their PCOS, and improve their health and well-being.

Physical activity and PCOS

By now you know Insulin Resistance and high insulin levels are significant features of PCOS.[5]

In a randomised study, young women with PCOS followed a three-month exercise program, with 30-minute structured exercise periods. These women experienced significant improvement in their levels of insulin sensitivity compared to those who remained sedentary.[6]

Exercise also increases antioxidant levels. Women with PCOS have been found to have increased oxidative stress and decreased antioxidant levels.[7,8]

Women with PCOS are more likely to develop anxiety and depression.[9,10] (It is well known that exercise improves mood, and decreases anxiety and depression.)

Women with PCOS are at more risk of cardiovascular conditions. A three-month Exercise Training (ET) program showed improved cardiopulmonary functional capacity in young women suffering from PCOS.[11]

Moderate walking programs helped minimise the risk of cardiovascular risk factors in overweight and obese women with PCOS.[12]

The University of Adelaide looked at the effect of a six-month diet and exercise program on 18 overweight women. They experienced amazing changes in their hormonal levels – 71% improvement in insulin sensitivity, 33% fall in the insulin levels, 39% reduction in luteinising hormone (LH) levels and 11% reduction in central fat.[13] Very exciting findings for a woman with PCOS.

The list goes on.

Exercises you can do

You need to start where you're at. It doesn't matter where this is, just begin moving. If you have been exercising regularly, great. If it's a long while since you've been active, or you are significantly overweight, a walk to the letter box may be enough in the beginning. Movement changes your joints, as does a lack of movement. Excessive weight strains your organs, your joints, your body. So, start sensibly. Obesity places more strain on your heart, so a gently, gently approach may be needed in the beginning.

As a Chiropractor I know once said to me: "You can't sprint a marathon". You may need to pace yourself. Physical activity needs to be ingrained in your lifestyle. A learning and adaptive process for your body and brain – not a chore. Remember, every step you take is improving your health, bringing you closer to your goal of conquering your PCOS, and helping you to achieve a vital body, mind and soul.

Here are some steps to help you increase your physical activity:

Learn to love activity!

Step 1: Remember why you are exercising. Your primary aim really should be to *get and stay well.* Write down your motivating ideas. Make them really personal. They need to be dear to your heart. Something to keep you going if times get hard. Look at these regularly.

Step 2: Just start. Do something. Get up off your chair or sofa. Just get moving!

Step 3: Add incidental exercise to your day. Sit on a Swiss ball instead of your desk chair, walk to the letterbox, to work, to the shops, to post your mail.

Step 4: Find what you love to do and do it. Don't do what you hate to do. There are always options that will make you light up. Do these. If you're a Zumba queen, then Zumba. Garden. If you love basketball, join a team. If you love to walk among the butterflies and flowers, find a local garden and do so.

Step 5: Have fun. If you love Pink, put her on your MP3 player, turn up the sound, and dance around the house to build up a sweat.

Step 6: Commit yourself. Get a personal trainer and agree to train on specific day/s and time/s. Join a team. Walk with a friend, maybe one who already has a walking routine.

Step 7: Build slowly. Remember, it has taken years for you to reach your current health status. It will take time to improve, for your body and your brain to change, and correctly adapt. Just put one foot in front of the other and keep moving.

Step 8: Once you reach your goal, and you are feeling healthy, vibrant and clear, keep going. Challenge yourself. Encourage others. Physical activity needs to be a lifelong habit.

What type of physical activity should you do?

What type of physical activity should you do? A variety.

You need to build your aerobic and anaerobic capacity; to build your muscles – those that make your limbs move, and those that support your spine, your body, your posture; you need to improve your proprioception (proprioception is your joint position sense and an important brain nutrient); and to healthily stretch your muscles, joints, ligaments and soft tissues. These different types of exercise will give your body what it needs for optimal health, while also improving your insulin sensitivity, and other components of PCOS.

A. Sweaty exercise

You know what I mean, the type of exercise that gets your heart pumping and skin sweating. If you are a little phobic about long, drawn out workouts, you are about to hear some very good news. You don't need to work out for long periods of time. You can get a better workout, in a shorter timeframe, by interval training. Dr Gail Trapp's research shows by doing eight seconds of high intensity work, followed by 12 seconds of relative rest, you use more fat as fuel.[14] Dr Babraj also looked at short duration, high intensity training. He found after only two weeks of training (which included six sessions, each with 4–6 cycle sprints of 30seconds), blood sugar levels improved dramatically.[15]

Imagine, you can improve your body's ability to control its blood sugar in only two weeks!

What does Dr Trapp and Dr Babraj's research tell us? You can make big improvements to your body in a short amount of time, if you train right. You can lose fat, improve your blood sugar control, and become healthier, faster with shorter training times.

Common types of exercise that you can incorporate a 'sprint' into include:

- Walking
- Jogging
- Running
- Swimming
- Cycling
- Rowing/kayaking

- Tennis/squash/other racquet sports (naturally include a sprint component)
- Cross training
- Dancing
- Skipping.

B. Resistance training

Resistance training (also called strength training) is vital for your well-being. We no longer climb trees or hills, or chase and wrestle our food or foes, so we need to add this type of movement into our lives. Resistance training is wonderful for improving your muscle and bone strength, posture, fat burning ability, coordination, insulin sensitivity, and our cardiovascular and neuro-musculoskeletal system.[16]

Resistance training is what we normally think of as 'going to the gym'. Weights machines are helpful, but I am a big fan of using free weights. Free weights use the specific muscles an exercise is designed for, plus those required to stabilise your body. This gives you a better work out, and works more muscles at one time. A mix of functional and free weight training is the best recommendation. What if you don't like, or can't afford to go to a gym? Easy, no excuses... buy or borrow some dumb bells, a Swiss ball, a theraband. Do pushups, wall pushups, crunches, squats, lunges, walking lunges, step-ups... the list goes on. Hold a food can, then lift, and you have overhead rows. For more ideas, simply search the internet.

TIP: Exercise until you feel that burn. Once you reach the level of lactic acid build up, you are well on your way to improving your hormonal profile.

C. Flexibility enhancing exercise

Stretching improves spinal movement, and lengthens your

muscles and ligaments. Modern day living involves too much sitting. This is not only inflammatory, but it causes our bodies, in essence, to become 'stuck' in unnatural postures. Stretching helps us get 'unstuck'. Stretching can be mixed with breathing and strengthening, and can even help you relax your mind. You can perform each of these individually, or get involved in an activity that incorporates many of these aspects.

Some great ways to stretch, improve flexibility, improve your posture, and learn to relax your body and brain are:

- Yoga
- Pilates
- T'ai Chi.

Practise Yoga

Yoga is the ancient Indian form of exercise. A very important benefit of Yoga to PCOS women is its ability to decrease your stress. Stress, as we discussed in Chapter 6, causes weight gain, infertility and disease. Yoga helps by training you to control your movements and muscles, tone your body, breathe correctly, and relax.

Chiropractic

> *"90% of the nutrition to the brain is generated by the movement of the spine"*
>
> *Dr Roger Sperry, M.D. (Nobel Prize Recipient for Brain Research)*

We have known for some time that a part of your brain, called your cerebellum, and your autonomic nervous system (ANS) have a very close relationship. Your ANS is the part of your nervous system that controls your fight-or-flight system (your sympathetic or stress system), and your relaxation system (your parasympathetic system). Although your cerebellum is relatively small compared to your brain, it contains within it more than half of the neurons in all of your nervous system.[17] This means your cerebellum is critically important in how you function.

Making up more than 50% of your spinal cord is something called your proprioceptive pathways. These are essential to your health, as proprioception is what energises your cerebellum, and so energises your brain.

From your cerebellum, to your hypothalamus. Remember, your hypothalamus is that vital gland with a significant role in controlling your hormone levels. As Dr James Chestnut puts it: "Proprioception from movement is relayed to the hypothalamus, which elicits immediate visceral motor responses."[18] This means movement literally changes the way your organs actually work, via your spine.

Your cerebellum affects your stress system, emotions, thoughts[19], movement and posture. It can even affect learning, performance and motivation[20], heart rate and blood pressure.

Why am I telling you about your cerebellum? What effect could this have on your PCOS? And why Chiropractic? It's simple. If your spinal joints aren't moving correctly, you are not receiving the proprioceptive signals you need to fully energise your brain. Worse than that, you are also receiving increased harmful, or noxious, stimulation (nociception). This is a nasty combination, and one that adversely affects your brain function.

Chiropractic adjustments[21] and exercise increase optimal brain function through increased proprioception. This optimal brain function is important for you in conquering your PCOS and is also absolutely essential if you are to reach optimal wellness. For more information about Chiropractic care, see *www.ConquerPCOSNaturally.com/Chiropractic*

A recent study offers sufficient evidence of the possibility of creating a complementary-care plan and an integrated wellness program of Yoga practice and Chiropractic care in the management of health issues.[22]

Posture

In our modern age, we constantly sit and stoop. This physically changes our spine, shortens and tightens some of our muscles, tendons, ligaments and fascia, while lengthening others. It stops the correct movement of our joints. We need to actively address our posture to improve our health. I discuss your posture in greater detail in the course available at *www.ConquerYourPCOSCourse.com*

The six golden rules of movement

Hopefully by now, you can see the importance of correct movement in overcoming your PCOS, and in attaining optimal health. Here are some tips to help you on your way:

- Start where you are. If you are very unfit, start very gently. If you have organs that don't work as well as they should, including your heart, you still need to start. If you have any health concerns, seek guidance and support from a supportive, qualified health care professional.

- Set concrete goals, be disciplined and reward yourself with something wonderful – other than food.

- Learn to listen to your body. If safe, push yourself. Also, get proper rest.

- Join an exercise group, a team, a gym, a Yoga class. Tee up movement time with a friend. Add in incidental exercise. Sweep the floors instead of vacuuming, lift each food tin in a shoulder press while putting it away. Start walking. Ride an exercise bike while watching television. Take the stairs instead of the lift.

- Find innovative ways to move. The same routine can be boring. Try dancing, hiking or stair-climbing.

- Find a Chiropractor, and get your spine checked regularly. Initially, you may need an intensive course of care. Once stable, you need a checkup once every 1–4 weeks, depending on your body and lifestyle. Your Chiropractor will be able to advise you on the best frequency for you. Remember, the most important reason to be under regular Chiropractic care is not for its effectiveness at pain relief, but for its wonderful ability to improve your brain function and so improve your health.

What are you waiting for? Get up and move!

Can't get enough?

Go to *www.ConquerYourPCOSNaturally.com/ BonusReports* to grab your FREE bonuses.

As an additional bonus, you'll also receive Dr Rebecca's *'Conquer Your PCOS'* monthly newsletter for FREE. You'll discover even more PCOS advice, easy-to-apply practical tips, PCOS-friendly recipes, and become a *'Conquer Your PCOS'* VIP.

Act now and join us and the 'Conquer Your PCOS' community!

Also, follow Dr Rebecca at:

www.Facebook.com/ConquerYourPCOS
and
http://Twitter.com/ConquerPCOS

Chapter Twelve

Your Ideal Weight

Finally, the secrets to weight loss for a woman with PCOS revealed! I've lost 20kg (that's 44 pounds) and you can too. If you're underweight, I discuss this too.

> *"In the Middle-Ages, they had guillotines, stretch racks, whips and chains. Nowadays, we have a much more effective torture device called the 'bathroom scale'."*
>
> Stephen Phillips

Whether you are underweight, your ideal weight or overweight, many women feel conscious of their size. So, what is your ideal weight? And why does how much you weigh really matter? We will address these questions throughout this chapter.

Among the multitude of different diets and society's lust for the size zero model, the concept of ideal weight – your healthy weight – seems to have become lost. For women with PCOS, reaching an ideal weight is often difficult.

The majority of women with PCOS are overweight or obese. However, this syndrome also affects women who are trim, or underweight. I will discuss both ends of the spectrum as it relates to PCOS.

Why is weight important?

Reaching your ideal weight will help rectify your Insulin

Resistance, rebalance your hormones, boost your ovulation and fertility[1] and overcome your PCOS.

Why fuss over fat?

Fat is not all bad. It is an essential body tissue. In fact, girls won't start menstruating until they reach 17% body fat.[2] You need a healthy amount of fat for normal menses, ovulation, optimal fertility and your general well-being. However, having too much body fat can result in irregular periods, anovulation, decreased fertility, increased 'male' hormone levels, poor self-esteem, Insulin Resistance and more. Having too little fat also affects our menstrual cycle, fertility and function.

Having an ideal amount of body fat is important. The following table provides a guide to what is normal. Consulting a personal trainer, specialised Naturopath or other qualified professional will help determine your fat percentage.

CLASSIFICATION	WOMEN (% FAT)	MEN (% FAT)
ESSENTIAL FAT	10 - 13%	2 - 5%
ATHLETES	14 - 20%	6 - 13%
FITNESS	21 - 24%	14 - 17%
AVERAGE	25 - 31%	18 - 24%
OBESE	32% and higher	25% and higher

http://www.acefitness.org/blog/112/what-are-the-guidelines-for-percentage-of-body-fat/#

What is body mass index (BMI)?

The risk of PCOS and the severity of its symptoms increase with increasing BMI. On one hand, where losing weight with an improved food plan and exercise restores fertility in overweight and obese women with PCOS, such a weight loss can be hazardous for fertility in lean women.[3]

Body mass index is a weight to height ratio used to help determine ideal weight. To calculate this, divide your weight in kilograms by your height in metres squared:

$$BMI = weight\ (kg)/height\ (m)^2$$

– or – multiply your weight in pounds by 703. Then divide this by your height in inches squared:

$$BMI = weight\ (lb)\ x\ 703/height\ (inches)^2$$

An ideal BMI falls between 20–25, although different sources give some variation on the lower end of this scale. For example, the chart below lists an ideal weight as a BMI above 18.5 (although this is not ideal for optimal fertility). BMI is by no means perfect for all people (i.e. athletes may falsely fall in the obese class, and it is not accurate in children or the elderly), however it is a good, simple indicator of healthy weight.

How else can you assess your size and risk of dis-ease?

Waist circumference is a good indicator of dis-ease risk. To measure your waist circumference, have someone help you. You need to stand comfortably, with your arms relaxed by your side. When the measurement is taken, your stomach is in a relaxed position, and you take a normal in breath. Your assistant lays a measuring tape snugly, but not tightly, around your waist. (To find your waist, let your elbow fall gently by your side. The crook of your elbow will be at the level of your waist.) The tape needs to be horizontal to the floor.

Once you have determined your weight, BMI and waist circumference, you can determine whether you need to lose weight, gain weight or maintain the weight you are currently.

Classification of overweight and obesity by BMI, waist circumference and associated dis-ease risk*

	BMI (kg/m²)	Obesity Class	Dis-ease Risk* Relative to Normal Weight and Waist Circumference	
			Men ≤ 102 cm (≤ 40 in) Women ≤ 88 cm (≤ 35 in)	> 102 cm (> 40 in) > 88 cm (> 35 in)
UNDERWEIGHT	**<18.5**	—	—	—
NORMAL+	**18.5-24.9**	—	—	—
OVERWEIGHT	**25.0-29.9**	—	**Increased**	**High**
OBESITY	**30.0-34.9**	**I**	**High**	**Very High**
	35.0-39.9	**II**	**Very High**	**Very High**
EXTREME OBESITY	**≥40**	**III**	**Extremely High**	**Extremely High**

* Dis-ease risk for type 2 diabetes, hypertension and cardiovascular dis-ease (CVD).

+ Increased waist circumference can also be a marker for increased risk even in persons of normal weight.

Source: www.nhlbi.nih.gov/guidelines/obesity/ob_gdlns.pdf

Secrets of reaching your 'ideal weight'

For many women with PCOS, weight loss attempts can be incredibly difficult, and many women believe after countless attempts, they are doomed to be overweight or obese forever. If successful in losing weight, their happiness is often short-lived. The weight, and often more, may rush back with a vengeance. Does this sound like you? There is some good news. In this chapter, we are going to reveal the secrets to not only losing weight, but keeping it off.

If you are underweight, we will walk you through the road less travelled, giving tips on food and physical activity to help you also reach your ideal weight.

I hope to shift your focus to achieving your 'ideal body weight' to ensure not only improved fertility and self-esteem, but to guide you down the road to optimal health and well-being.

What is your motivation?

The first thing I want you to do, regardless of whether you wish to lose or gain weight, is write down the three major reasons you wish to change your body weight for the better. Make these really personal, emotional. They should bring a tear to your eye. Keep these handy. Look at these daily. If there is a time when you are feeling low, or you have temporarily stepped off the bandwagon, read these, out loud. Repeat. Know why you are making these changes toward optimal health.

Losing weight and gaining health

"Losing weight comes down to calories in versus calories out." I'm sure you've been told this before?

Consuming more calories than you use is certainly one factor in weight gain. When you wish to lose weight, you need to use more than you take in. But, there is much more to this story. If you have consulted a professional to try to lose weight previously, you have most likely been told 'it is all about less energy coming in and more energy going out'. Many women with PCOS are told this – and no more – over and over again. They leave the consultation feeling depressed, unheard, with a sense of failure and confusion. Scratching their heads and wondering. They know they don't eat as much as some of their slender friends and yet the kilograms keep piling on. Despite the low calorie, low sugar, low fat, high protein, lemon detox, alternate day diet… you still can't lose weight… *why?*

Myths and facts about starving and 'low calorie' diets busted

If you've thought about or have been starving yourself to get thin, or have used laxatives or forced yourself to vomit, you are not alone. Desperate attempts to lose weight have pushed women with PCOS towards serious eating disorders. Women with PCOS are at an increased risk of 'bulimia' (an eating disorder where a person binge eats and then throws up deliberately or uses laxatives to purge the food).[4]

The never-ending cycle of desperate attempts at losing weight and guilt over not being able to do so, may trap you in a painful situation tainted with guilt, shame and disappointment.

There may be reasons why a very low calorie diet (eating less than 800 calories a day) seems appealing. However, although emotionally it may seem a logical step, it is not only unsustainable, it is very bad for you.

Starving is bad for your thyroid

When your body is repeatedly starved of calories, it can upset the balance of your thyroid gland (remember from Chapter 9 this gland controls the energy level of your body). Due to low energy reserves, the thyroid gland reduces the conversion of T4 to the active T3 hormone. There may also be an increase in levels of inactive reverse T3. All this leads to a lowering of the function of your thyroid. This hypothyroid situation can make it difficult for you to lose weight. Adding to your weight loss woes, this condition may make you put on more weight.[5]

Starving starves your muscles

Low calorie diets starve your body of the vital energy and nutrients needed to sustain health. To compensate for this energy shortage, your body may start using your muscle tissue as energy. This precious muscle mass is important in helping you burn energy. Even though you may initially shed kilograms on the scales, it is not the harmful fat you are losing, but health-giving lean muscle.

Loss of muscle mass means loss of muscle tone. You look flabbier, and you lose your ability to efficiently burn fat.

Eating less can cause toxin build up

Fat cells are the safest place to store toxins unable to be removed from your body. When we begin to lose weight, these toxins are released into our bodies. You need ample nutrients to detoxify safely and fully. If you are eating a very restrictive diet, you will not have the nutritional reserves to effectively remove these toxins. Toxins can cause a cascade of imbalances, from decreasing your insulin sensitivity, to inhibiting your weight loss.

A stressed heart

Very low calorie diets have been shown to create arterial stress. The combination of ineffective long-term weight loss attempts and stress on your cardiovascular system is a very unhealthy mix.

Do you have an unhealthy relationship with food?

As we just discussed, women with PCOS are at an increased

risk of bulimia[6], which is described as an eating disorder characterised by episodes of secretive excessive eating (binge-eating) followed by inappropriate methods of weight control, such as self-induced vomiting (purging), abuse of laxatives and diuretics, or excessive exercise.[34]

If you suspect you may have an eating disorder (symptoms like perpetual lack of hunger, compulsive vomiting episodes after eating or laxative use) seek professional help immediately. Eating disorders are dangerous and may be life threatening. If needed, professional help (psychotherapy and cognitive behavioural therapy) should be sought[7] sooner rather than later. The support of understanding loved ones can be priceless when faced with such a challenge.

The lesson I hope you've learnt is *never starve yourself* in an attempt to lose weight!

How can you lose weight?

Lifestyle change is the only way to truly overcome your PCOS, regain your health and effectively lose – and maintain – your optimal weight.

Let's begin with food.

Before you make any changes, I

> ### *Fast food versus slow food:*
>
> *Fast foods aren't fast just because they can be made in a jiffy. They are high in carbohydrate, often low in fibre, and so are digested FAST. They cause fast and significant spikes in your blood sugar and insulin levels. This contributes to blood sugar fluctuations and Insulin Resistance.*
>
> *'Slow foods' such as fruits like apples, salad and vegetables are rich in complex carbohydrates, fibre and nutrients. They are digested slowly and create slow and sustained blood sugar levels.*
>
> *When it comes to food, choose 'slow foods'.*

recommend you keep a food diary. Write down everything that goes in your mouth – food and drink. Track your intake for a minimum of three days, including the time. Also, note how you are feeling, any cravings and/or any symptoms. This will give you an honest idea of what you take in and when, and will give valuable insight into how the foods you eat make you feel, which foods are your weakness and when, and which foods in particular may cause you concern.

Get the right kind of carbohydrate, protein and fat

The most potent way to improve your insulin sensitivity is by the food and drink you consume, and those you don't. Insulin Resistance is a major driver in PCOS, and the exciting news is the healthy function of this critical hormone is under your control. Improving your insulin sensitivity helps you to achieve healthy weight loss and maintain your ideal weight.

A food plan that is low in simple carbohydrates, contains healthy proteins and healthy fats, plus the nutrients required for your body to function optimally, will aid in weight loss, while helping you to conquer your PCOS.

Choosing the right carbohydrate, in the right amount

Removing carbohydrates which offer no nutritional value and cause your insulin levels to increase is essential for weight loss in PCOS. Foods such as sugar, flour, bread, pasta, potatoes, processed and packaged foods, soft drinks and packaged fruit juices, biscuits, cakes and lollies should be removed from your food plan. Keep reading for some good news about chocolate.

Choose your carbs smartly from salads, fruits and vegetables with a healthy low glycaemic load. Also, remember that the amount of energy your body needs is proportional to the amount of physical activity you do. That is, if you live a sedentary lifestyle, your body needs fewer calories than if you live an active life.

- Eliminate breads, pasta, bagels, muffins, biscuits and white rice from your diet.
- Let your snacks be fresh fruits and vegetables, boiled eggs, nuts, salad or tuna.
- Purge your pantry and refrigerator of sugary treats, drinks, condiments and sweets. Make a pact with yourself. If you 'have to have' that chocolate bar, you will walk to the shop to buy it.
- Do not eat carbohydrates for your evening meal. This will help reduce higher blood sugar levels overnight. You don't want to put on weight while you are sleeping.
- Don't let yourself become hungry. Eat smaller meals more regularly. Include a healthy morning and afternoon snack.
- If you are experiencing uncontrollable cravings, first go for a 10-minute walk. Eat a salad first. If you still want it, eat it slowly, consciously. Smell it thoroughly. Move it around your mouth and feel the texture. Don't feel guilty. As you go through this journey, these cravings will subside.

How much is enough carbohydrate?

When you are wishing to lose weight, you must weigh up not only the quickest way forward, but also your ability to stick with the food plan. Initially, a very low carbohydrate (ketogenic) food plan is very effective. Plans that include below 30–60 grams of carbohydrates daily have been shown to yield impressive fat and weight loss[8], while preserving muscle mass. Studies show a very low carbohydrate food plan (less than 30 grams per day) resulted in higher body weight lost, and higher weight lost as fat.[9] If you feel you can no longer sustain a very low carbohydrate food plan, you may switch to a relatively higher carbohydrate food plan (approximately 60–100 grams per day). This will still result in weight loss, just at a slower pace.

Decreasing your carbohydrate intake and increasing your healthy protein consumption results in more fat loss than high carbohydrate diets.[10] Lower carbohydrate food plans also keep you feeling full longer.[11]

Once you have reached your ideal weight, following a similar plan but including more healthy carbohydrates such as gluten-free whole grains, more healthy protein and more fruits will allow you to maintain your weight and also your health. There are other health benefits to a lower carbohydrate eating plan. One study found a lower carbohydrate, high-protein food plan improved not only weight loss, and weight lost as fat in women with PCOS, it also resulted in larger decreases in serum cholesterol.[12]

A balanced low-carbohydrate food plan is safe. If you find yourself constipated, ensure you are including enough leafy green vegetables, salad and appropriate vegetables such as artichoke, capsicum, broccoli, cauliflower and cucumber. For a detailed list of appropriate vegetables, see Chapter 17 'Eat your way to health – The best food plan to conquer your PCOS'. Reducing or eliminating starchy vegetables such as potatoes is also helpful.

A ketogenic food plan causes formation of ketone bodies. These can be measured by a strip known as a 'ketostix'. When you are following this type of food plan, testing your urine with a ketostix morning and night will let you know if you are eating the right amount of carbohydrate. Ketostix are inexpensive, and should be available from your local chemist or specialised health care professional.

Benefits of a ketogenic food plan:

- Improves metabolic syndrome – decreases total cholesterol and triglycerides, and blood sugar levels, and increases HDL levels.[13]

- Is effective at fat reduction, while maintaining healthy muscle mass and hydration.[14]
- Improves irritable bowel syndrome.[15]
- Suits the metabolic needs of women with PCOS.
- Decreases cravings.

NOTE: If you are a type 1 diabetic, please seek professional assistance before embarking on this type of food plan. You may be better suited to a Mediterranean-style eating plan.

TIP: Aside from helping you lose weight, a very low carbohydrate diet has been shown to improve irritable bowel syndrome (IBS).[16]

Increase your healthy proteins

When I say increase your protein intake, I do not mean loading up with unhealthy burgers, fried sausages and bucket loads of cheese. The type of protein included makes a big difference to your health. Including plenty of healthy proteins in your food plan helps your weight loss. Including lean sources of proteins with a preference for plant-based, seafood and organic eggs is important. Plant-based proteins are healthy and well-suited to the metabolic needs of women with PCOS.

Eggs, nuts such as almonds and walnuts, and seeds like pumpkin seeds and flaxseeds are good sources of protein. Add them to your salads or make your own trail mix by choosing from a wide variety of nuts and seeds. Including fish (steamed, curried, lightly grilled) is also a healthy way of increasing the healthy proteins in your food plan.

The perks of increasing your protein intake include:

- Aids in maintaining your lean muscle mass. This helps you burn energy more effectively.
- Helps in lowering the risk of diabetes, hypertension, heart dis-ease and cancers like lung and colon cancer.[17]

- Protein increases our feeling of fullness and lengthens the time we feel full.

- One study showed as more protein was eaten, people naturally decreased the amount of food they ate. An increase in protein intake was even shown to decrease the amount of calories eaten by people who were allowed to choose what they ate. This helps with weight loss.[18]

Fat fundamentals

As strange as it seems, you need a steady supply of good fats in order to lose unwanted fat. Fats are essential building blocks for normal hormone production, including those involved in reproductive function; they help us use vitamins, are critical for our brain and nervous system and for healthy skin, they provide energy, are anti-inflammatory, insulin sensitising and they allow our cells to communicate. In fact, every cell in our body needs fats to be well. Without healthy fats in your food plan, you can't be well either. Neither can you lose weight effectively or healthily, or conquer your PCOS.

However, all fats are not created equal. In modern society, we have an imbalance of omega-6:omega-3 fats. This imbalance favours omega-6 fats and inflammation, which favours weight gain. Fast foods, baked products, packaged foods and more, use partially hydrogenated oils (trans fats). These trans fats have been linked to cardiovascular dis-ease (CVD)[19], diabetes[20], obesity[21], infertility[22] and depression.[23] These health challenges are a concern in themselves, but can also affect your ability to lose weight (i.e. depression leads to a lack of motivation, and CVD, diabetes and obesity can curtail how you exercise).

Obese people also have a greater preference for fat-rich foods, and resort more often to comfort eating.[24] Excessive intake of unhealthy fat can decrease your insulin sensitivity, cause imbalances in your hormone production, interfere with ovulation, increase your risk of heart dis-ease and, of course, make you heavier.

Benefits of fat in weight loss

- Omega-3 fats such as those in fish oil, halibut, trout, walnuts, flaxseed oil and shrimp reduce inflammation, improve insulin sensitivity, and in conjunction with exercise, have been shown to boost fat loss.[25]

Acidic and alkaline foods[26]

ACID-PRODUCING FOODS	ALKALINE-PRODUCING FOODS	NEUTRAL FOODS
CEREAL GRAINS - Rice, Wheat, Oats	Nuts and Seeds+, Walnuts and Walnut Oil, Flaxseeds, Pumpkin Seeds	Legumes
MEAT	Fresh Fruit	
POULTRY	Tubers like: Sweet Potato, Yam, Cassava (Yuca)	
MILK	Mushrooms+	
SHELLFISH	Vegetables+	
CHEESE	Leafy Greens+	
	Quinoa and Buckwheat	

+*Particularly valuable in a weight loss plan*

Ensuring alkalinity (or base)

A ketogenic food plan can increase acidity in the body. To balance this, and maintain health while still being in a fat-burning state, foods such as leafy green vegetables and low glycaemic fruits and vegetables need to be included.

You can measure your pH while on a ketogenic food plan by performing urinary pH testing. Your pH should be between 6.5–7.5. pH strips are inexpensive and quick to use, and should be available from your local chemist or specialised health care professional. Checking your pH weekly is sufficient.

How much to eat?

Our portion sizes have expanded massively (often, more than doubled) in the past 20 years. So much so that it's hard to recognise what 'normal' actually is. Greater portion size means greater energy intake, and this means growing waist lines.

To tailor your portion size for your weight loss needs, simply use the 'palm method'. Here are some 'rules of palm' that will help you choose the right amount of food for you:

- Each meal should be made of three rounded handfuls of vegetables/salad plus one palm sized portion (your palm size in width, length and depth) of lean, healthy protein.

- You should have two daily snacks of healthy protein equal to approximately the size of your second, third and fourth fingers combined.

- You should include 1–2 tablespoons of healthy oils, a three-finger portion of nuts, or a serve of oily fish daily.

NOTE: You can replace one handful of salad per day with one handful of allowable fruit (see Chapter 17 'Eat your way to health – The best food plan to conquer your PCOS'). Many women find it easier to use meal replacements in addition to other weight-loss measures. This can be a valuable addition, but please ensure the company you purchase these from is health conscious, ethical and knowledgeable, and that their products are toxin-free.

Experiment with your culinary skills. For recipe ideas see 'Conquer Your PCOS – 50+ Delicious & Healthy Recipes for Optimal Living' at *www.ConquerYourPCOSNaturally.com/OtherBooks*

Supplement solutions

Without the necessary nutrients, your body will be unable to successfully lose fat. Here are some nutrients that can assist you in your weight loss, and protect your health during this critical transition:

- EPA/DHA (fish oil). (Vegetarians can use flaxseed oil)
- Coenzyme Q10
- L-carnitine
- Calcium, chromium, magnesium, selenium
- Vitamins D, C and E
- Pre and probiotics
- Multivitamins and minerals.

Secrets of a successful transition to a healthier, slimmer you

- Keep a food diary to help you assess your food and liquid intake, particularly in the beginning. Not only can you keep an honest eye on what is being put in your mouth, but you can ensure there is variety in your food plan, and that enough fresh fruit and vegetables are being consumed.
- Purchase a smaller plate to eat from and don't return for seconds.
- Get help and support from your loved ones. Your emotions can play a big role when it comes to weight loss. See Chapter 16 'Communicate Well – A guide for your loved ones to understand and support you' for some more tips.
- Join a weight-loss or health group to help you stay motivated. Having someone you are accountable to can help you in your weight loss.

- Beat your stress. A chronically stressed you is a heavier you! Yoga, meditation, T'ai Chi, regular Chiropractic care, massage, aromatherapy and so forth are great for relieving stress. For more information and tips on stress, see Chapter 6 'Stress - Learn how to beat stress, rediscover happiness, regain your focus and get your mojo back'

- Buy some 'Ketostix' – these sticks are very useful. Placed in your urinary stream, they allow you to see if you are in the 'fat burning zone'.

- Drink like a fish. Drinking a minimum of eight glasses of pure water daily aids weight loss, increases calories burnt, and can help you feel full.

- Drink green tea.

- Include low carbohydrate, higher protein morning and afternoon snacks.

- Get up and move! Encourage weight loss by improving your metabolic rate and lean muscle mass, decreasing your stress and using more calories. Maintain an adequate and safe exercise routine. Remember – when it comes to exercise, it is not only the amount, but the continuity and persistence that matters.

- Ensure you receive enough sleep.

- If you hit a plateau, consider a healthy and safe detoxification program. Toxins can limit or halt weight loss.

- Be aware of any self-sabotaging behaviours. For some women, being a certain weight provides an underlying benefit (i.e. being bigger may subconsciously make you feel safer). If you need to, seek counselling. Positive affirmations may help.

- Identify eating triggers. Avoid these if possible, and put in place alternatives.

- Addressing all the factors affecting fat loss may require professional help. Factors include stress, low thyroid function, inflammation, acidic pH, a leaky gut, toxicity, and hormonal imbalance.[27]

Last but not least, an indulgent tip. For those of you who enjoy a little bit of chocolate, there is some good news. A small amount of chocolate once a week may decrease your risk of heart dis-ease, and encourage weight loss. The smell of chocolate may even aid weight loss. The proviso – it needs to be dark chocolate, and only a small amount. Clear your calendar, ensure some quiet time. Sit down with your favourite cup of hot herbal tea, and your piece of chocolate. Take a deep breath, smell. Gently place the chocolate in your mouth, let it melt a little. Slowly does it. Enjoy!

Are you underweight?

A lot less is said about the woes of women who suffer with PCOS and have a less than ideal body mass index (BMI) (BMI <20). Despite their thin appearance, these women often still have Insulin Resistance, higher 'male' hormones, menstrual irregularities and infertility. Lean women with PCOS were shown to have a higher body fat percentage and lower lean body mass (muscle) when compared with age- and weight-matched women without PCOS.[28]

Lean women with PCOS have higher blood androgen levels than women without PCOS.[29] These higher levels of 'male' hormone levels were decreased by sensitising these women to insulin.[30]

Conceiving a child may be equally as challenging for lean women with PCOS as for those women who are overweight. Even if conception occurs, there is a higher risk of their babies being born with a low birth weight. Lower BMI also lowers the chance of success when using assisted reproductive treatments like *in vitro* fertilisation (IVF).[31]

If you have lost weight suddenly or quickly, seek professional help. Some conditions can cause weight loss such as hyperthyroidism, depression, chronic diarrhoea, drug abuse and medications.

Reaching your ideal weight

Gaining weight for slender women can be equally as tough as losing it is for overweight women. Reaching the ideal BMI for fertility of 22–24 is crucial for reproductive health in women – to be able to conceive and deliver a healthy child. Research shows that increasing BMI with proper guidance leads to pregnancy and normal menstruation in up to 73% of women who are thin and suffer with PCOS.[32]

Food details

Writing down what you eat on a daily basis can help you determine if you are eating enough to maintain a healthy weight.

The food plan required to safely and healthily gain weight is still similar to those trying to lose weight. As lean women with PCOS often have Insulin Resistance and higher 'male' hormones, your food plan still needs to address these issues. When looking to gain weight, *calories in* versus *calories out* does matter.

- Regularly include healthy fats such as avocado and nuts. These healthy fats help you to overcome your PCOS, but also add calories.

- Keeping your Insulin Resistance in mind, you need to include low glycaemic carbohydrates regularly. Think fruits, vegetables and gluten-free grains.

- Proteins help in building muscle mass, hence including plenty of healthy protein is a must. Organic eggs and poultry, fresh fish and nuts are essential.

- Eat more regularly. This will allow you to increase the amount of calories you take in, without feeling 'stuffed', while maintaining healthy blood sugar levels.

- Avoid drinking fluids with your meals. Fluids contribute to a feeling of fullness, so not drinking with your meals means you can eat more.

- Add healthy smoothies.

TIP: Do not indulge in unhealthy foods full of sugar, additives and harmful fats. Although they will help you to gain weight, these foods are detrimental to your blood sugars, insulin levels, testosterone levels and your PCOS.

Are you stressed?

Although it is more common for people under stress to increase the amount of food they eat, in some women, stress has the opposite effect. This decreased food intake can result in weight loss. It is more likely for an already underweight woman to under eat during stress.[33,34] Focusing on stress reduction can not only help you in reaching your ideal weight but has many other advantages, such as improving insulin sensitivity[35], mood, fertility and general health.

Increase your physical activity

You need to move in order to be healthy and to conquer your PCOS. Building muscle helps you gain weight. Good muscle tone is critical to health. Resistance training is important to build muscle. Cardiovascular exercise is important for health and well-being, so do not neglect this. However, overdoing this may lead to weight loss.

Are you your ideal weight already?

Great! Check your waist circumference as well as your BMI. Normal weight women with PCOS can still carry too much weight around their middle, and this is the most dangerous place to carry fat. Also, having your body fat percentage measured is a valuable indicator. The above points a still very relevant to you. You must follow a lower carbohydrate food plan in order to maintain healthy insulin levels. This eating plan will also help you reduce high testosterone, increase Sex Hormone Binding Globulin, reduce excessive oestrogen levels, boost optimal muscle mass, reduce stress and conquer your PCOS.

Whether you are looking to lose weight, gain weight or maintain your ideal weight, being your optimal body weight is a critical step in conquering your PCOS. When times get hard, look back to what motivates you. If you temporarily fall off the horse, take a breath and get back on. If you lost that horse a long while ago, let me help you find it. With lifestyle changes and a little effort, it is possible to achieve a lasting, healthy body weight. Remember...

"Some people dream about success...
while others wake up and work hard at it."

Winston Churchill

Can't get enough?

Go to *www.ConquerYourPCOSNaturally.com/BonusReports* to grab your FREE bonuses.

As an additional bonus, you'll also receive Dr Rebecca's *'Conquer Your PCOS'* monthly newsletter for FREE. You'll discover even more PCOS advice, easy-to-apply practical tips, PCOS-friendly recipes, and become a *'Conquer Your PCOS'* VIP.

Act now and join us and the 'Conquer Your PCOS' community!

Also, follow Dr Rebecca at:

www.Facebook.com/ConquerYourPCOS
and
http://Twitter.com/ConquerPCOS

Chapter Thirteen

Boost Your Fertility

Learn how to increase your chances of not only becoming pregnant, but carrying your healthy baby safely through to term

Why me? Facts on infertility in PCOS

Infertility is perhaps the biggest struggle experienced by women who suffer from PCOS.[1] Ninety to 95% of women who attend infertility clinics because of anovulation suffer from PCOS.[2] The challenges that PCOS causes in a woman's reproductive life do not end with just infertility. Those women who are fortunate to conceive despite having PCOS face a legion of complications that can jeopardise their own health and the health of their precious baby. Thirty to 50% of women with PCOS suffer miscarriages in the first trimester (first three months) of their pregnancy.[3] They may also have a greater risk for complications such as:

> *"It is said that if you know your enemies and know yourself, you will not be imperilled in a hundred battles."*
>
> **Sun Tzu, Great Chinese Military Strategist and the Author of The Art of War, 6th Century BC**

- Pregnancy induced hypertension (i.e. abnormally high blood pressure during pregnancy).
- Gestational diabetes (i.e. diabetes brought on by pregnancy).

- Preterm delivery (i.e. delivery before the completion of 37 weeks gestation).

Research studies also document a higher rate of neonatal intensive care (NICU) admissions of babies born to PCOS mothers due to post-delivery complications, as compared to those born to women without PCOS.[4] Although scary, these facts can help you to think about a strategy in advance – to face these challenges before they manifest, to not wait until it is too late. Your crusade against PCOS can seem like nothing less than a war. But, by educating yourself about every aspect of PCOS, you can take infertility, and its complications, head on to secure a healthy future for yourself and your baby.

How are PCOS, infertility and pregnancy complications related?

The imbalance of several hormones is the main reason for the infertility and pregnancy complications associated with PCOS. Let's review some of the various mechanisms that come into play.

High levels of luteinising hormone (LH)

High levels of the hormone LH is a common finding in women with PCOS. High levels of LH and an abnormal LH to Follicle Stimulating Hormone (FSH) ratio contribute to anovulation (failure in the maturation and release of eggs from the ovaries) in women with PCOS. In the absence of ovulation, infertility is unavoidable. Some studies also suggest that high levels of LH during certain stages of the menstrual cycle may prevent conception and even lead to early miscarriage. Even for women who opt for expensive assisted reproductive technologies (ART) like *in vitro* fertilisation (IVF), high levels of LH may be the main reason for poor treatment outcomes, low pregnancy rates and miscarriage.[5]

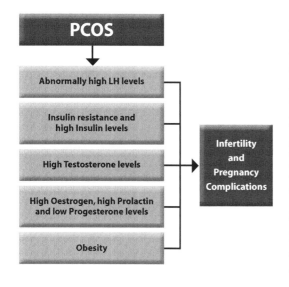

High insulin levels, high testosterone levels and insulin resistance

High insulin levels and Insulin Resistance are thought to trigger a number of hormonal imbalances in PCOS, the biggest one being an increased production of androgens like testosterone. The cumulative effect of this imbalance is infertility due to failure of the eggs to reach maturity, and anovulation.

Also, Insulin Resistance and high insulin levels (hyperinsulinemia) are the main cause of the development of 'gestational diabetes' in about 46% of pregnant women with PCOS.[6] Gestational diabetes can lead to 'macrosomia', or babies larger than normal newborns in terms of size and weight. Macrosomia increases the risk of trauma to the child during birth and the chances of a Caesarian section or C-section delivery.

TIP: Chiropractic care throughout pregnancy has been shown to decrease back pain during pregnancy and labour, and decrease labour time and pain.[7] A nervous system that functions optimally is invaluable. A body that functions optimally is better able to hold and deliver a baby.

Insulin Resistance can contribute to you piling on the kilograms during pregnancy, and can make these additional kilograms difficult to shed after delivery. Obesity associated with PCOS is yet another major factor that contributes to gestational diabetes during pregnancy.[8]

Obesity and Insulin Resistance are also two of the main factors associated with the development of pregnancy-induced hypertension (PIH) in women with PCOS. These two factors, along with physical inactivity, increase your risk for developing hypertension during pregnancy. PIH can have devastating effects and is one of the major causes behind pregnancy related health emergencies, potentially even causing maternal or foetal death.[9]

TIP: Magnesium helps to normalise blood pressure. Adding healthy foods naturally high in magnesium and a supplement can be most beneficial. Foods high in magnesium include red meat, turkey, chicken, nuts, sesame seeds, tahini, sunflower seeds, legumes, passionfruit, raspberries and bananas.

Oestrogen and progesterone imbalance

The state of oestrogen dominance (as discussed in Chapter 3 'Restore Your Hormonal Balance – Discover what your hormones do, how they affect your PCOS and the secrets to balancing them once more') creates a scenario of insufficient progesterone to balance oestrogen levels. A deficiency of progesterone, which is the hormone responsible for creating a favourable and fertile environment in the womb, can contribute to infertility. Additionally, an imbalance between oestrogen and progesterone levels lead to a change in the Hypothalamic-Pituitary-Gonadal (HPG) axis – the way your brain and reproductive organs talk to each other. This can cause anovulation and menstrual cycle disturbances, escalating the problem of infertility associated with PCOS.

Double check the cause of your infertility

Although PCOS is the leading cause of anovulatory infertility and subfertility, there are several other factors that may be affecting your ability to conceive. PCOS may be the obvious suspect, but you should also remember that there may be other factors contributing to your infertility.[10] If you are over the age of 35 and have been trying for six months or more, or under the age of 35 and have been trying for a year, you and your partner should consider consulting a specialist to zero in on the exact cause of your infertility. Forty per cent of the time, infertility is a result of female factors, 40% of the time, it's related to male factors and 20% of the time, the diagnosis is considered unknown.

Some other causes of infertility in women include:

Physical causes:

- Blockage of fallopian tubes due to infections, like pelvic inflammatory disease or Chlamydia.

- Endometriosis is a condition where cells of the endometrium, or uterine lining, abnormally migrate on to adjoining structures like the fallopian tubes, the tissues lining the pelvis (peritoneum), or the ovaries. This can lead to blockages, adhesions and cysts like the chocolate cyst of the ovary.

- Physical abnormalities of the uterus.

- Uterine fibroids, which are non-cancerous clumps of tissue and muscle on and in the walls of the uterus.[11]

Age:

The rate of infertility increases as you get older, especially above 35 years of age. This is because your stock – your number – of eggs begins to dwindle with age. Your body's ability to nourish a baby can diminish as you progress towards menopause. In women who use infertility treatments, like IVF, the chances of conceiving and having a successful and healthy pregnancy are significantly reduced in older women.[12] However, older women, don't despair. The type of lifestyle we encourage throughout this book can help increase the quality of your eggs, your fertility and your ability to respond to fertility medication, should you choose to go that route.

> *The rate of infertility in women according to their age is:*
>
> *8%: 19–26 years of age*
>
> *13-14%: 27–34 years of age*
>
> *18%: 35–39 years of age*
>
> Increased Infertility With Age in Men and Women, *by Dunson, David B., Baird, Donna D., Colombo, Bernardo,* Obstetrics & Gynecology, *January 2004, Volume 103 Issue 1, pp51–56.*

Smoking:

The general health hazards of smoking are well-known, but did you know that smoking can affect your fertility too? The increased number of women who smoke is one of the reasons behind the reduced fertility rates observed in the past 10 years. Smoking more than one pack of cigarettes per day, and starting to smoke before 18 years of age can both decrease your fertility.[13] Apart from the other deadly consequences associated with smoking, do you really want to be suddenly faced with concerns for your unborn child should you find yourself pregnant?

Alcohol:

There is no consensus in the medical community about the so called 'safe' level of alcohol consumption in women who want to conceive or those who are pregnant. Alcohol can have devastating effects both before, as well as after, conception. Even in 'moderate' amounts, alcohol consumption can contribute to first trimester spontaneous abortions[14], placental disruption[15], and future anxiety and depression in the growing baby.[16]

In my opinion, the only safe amount of alcohol during pregnancy is none. So ladies, for your own safety and that of your unborn baby – give up the booze.[17]

Caffeine:

Drinking more than two cups of coffee a day can be problematic if you are already struggling with infertility. Excessive caffeine intake has been linked to infertility and early miscarriage in women. Caffeine abuse before and during pregnancy can also lead to low birth weight babies.[18]

Street drugs:

Apart from the obvious detrimental effects of illicit drugs on your health, if you are looking to fall pregnant, street drugs simply must not be a part of the equation.

Marijuana can suppress Luteinising Hormone, and interfere with the luteal phase of the menstrual cycle.[19]

Heroin can result in an irregular menstrual cycle, and amenorrhea – the result of its suppressive effects on the hormones of the pituitary gland.[20]

Cocaine may have direct effects on the ovaries.[21]

Stress:

Your fertility depends greatly on the state of your mind. Mental and spiritual balance plays a pivotal role in conceiving a pregnancy. Research has shown that in women who are undergoing infertility treatment, high stress levels (manifested in feelings of depression, anxiety and being overwhelmed) and the associated high cortisol levels are related to poor pregnancy outcomes.[22] Chronic stress also interferes with GNrH production – a hormone whose production stimulates the release of LH and FSH, and is so crucial in your fertility.[23]

Stress can also adversely affect the growth of your baby. If you have high levels of cortisol while pregnant, this places both you and your growing baby, in the 'fight or flight response' (see Chapter 6 'Stress – Learn how to beat stress, rediscover happiness, regain your focus and get your mojo back'). In *Biology of Belief,* Dr Bruce Lipton refers to research showing that maternal stress can actually change the foetal blood distribution from the forebrain and organs, to the hindbrain and muscles. This can adversely affect your baby's stress (HPA) system, and potentially even their IQ.

Inflammation:

Inflammation adversely impacts fertility. Women with PCOS have been shown to have low grade inflammation, as measured by C-reactive protein (CRP)[24,25] and interleukin-6 (IL-6).

Another marker of inflammation – tumour necrosis factor (TNF) – is also elevated in women with PCOS[26] and in people who are obese.[27]

IL-6 stimulates the stress system and this suppresses the reproductive system. TNF also correlates with poor quality eggs.[28]

Thyroid:

An underactive thyroid may cause infrequent periods or periods with a very light flow (oligomenorrhoea), or excessive and prolonged bleeding (menorrhagia). An abnormal period may impact on fertility.[29]

An overactive thyroid gland (hyperthyroidism) results in "an increased risk of miscarriage, spontaneous abortion, foetal growth retardation, premature labour and delivery, congenital malformations and possibly pre-eclampsia".[30]

Read Chapter 9 'Your Thyroid – How to boost your metabolism, have abundant energy and lose weight' to learn more about your thyroid, and how to improve its function.

Nutrition:

Deficiency of vitamins and minerals like vitamins B12 and E, folate, iron and zinc, can be detrimental in women trying to conceive.[31] Crash dieting in the desperate hope of losing weight can easily cause nutrient deficiencies. Taking a daily prenatal vitamin and mineral, and eating a healthy diet will assist you in receiving sufficient amounts of the required nutrition.

> *Research conducted at the Harvard Medical School concluded there is a definite link between the amount of trans fat in a woman's diet and infertility. These fats are found in packaged, processed and baked foods. Avoid foods with 'partially hydrogenated vegetable oil'.*[35]

Sexually transmitted infections:

Certain sexually transmitted infections, like *Chlamydia trachomatis,* may be the hidden culprit behind your infertility.[32] It is also a significant reason for the failure of some fertility treatments. *C. trachomatis* infects the inner portion of the cervical canal called the 'endocervix', and can move up into the rest of the reproductive tract.

This infection can be silent with no apparent symptoms, although some women experience painful urination and a yellow green vaginal discharge. When your doctor performs a pap smear, ask him or her to also take cervical cultures for Chlamydia and other infections. These bacteria can hide up high in the cervix, so you need to have a high cervical swab taken.

pH:

Our systemic pH should be between 6.5–7.5. If the woman's cervical mucus is too acidic, the sperm are immobilised.

This means the sperm won't reach and fertilise the egg. Your cervical mucus is a reflection of your body's pH. As such, you can test this with a urinary pH test. You should be able to buy one from your local chemist. To increase the alkalinity of your mucus, follow the food plan recommended in this book (drink plenty of pure water, eliminate foods such as flour, white breads, sugar, pasta, alcohol and tobacco and increase your greens, fruits and vegetables, and healthy fats).

Get ready to make a baby

"Hold your head high, stick your chest out. You can make it. It gets dark sometimes, but morning comes. Keep hope alive."

Jesse Jackson

Truly, the times may seem very dark when you are suffering from PCOS. Infertility can feel devastating. However, channelling your efforts in the right direction can help hoist you out of this abyss. The first step forward is to understand your body and how it works to create and support a pregnancy.

Conceiving and nurturing offspring is a basic human instinct. Our body has such an amazing ability to prepare itself for a potential pregnancy every month. This process is called the menstrual cycle and is also known as the ovarian or reproductive cycle. As the name suggests, our menstrual cycle follows a repetitive pattern of hormonal activity along with corresponding ovarian and uterine changes every month. Our fertility depends on the normalcy of our menstrual cycle.

At least 60–80% of women suffering from PCOS have less than nine periods a year.[33] Many have even less. By understanding the phases of a normal cycle, you can appreciate the abnormalities in your own cycle. This will help you identify the steps you need to take in order to ensure a healthy reproductive cycle and, of course, a healthy baby.

The healthy menstrual cycle

The length of this cycle may vary from woman to woman. A normal cycle can be anywhere between 28 to 35 days long.[34] In a cycle of 28 days, these are the changes that take place in your body:

Day 1 to 13

FOLLICULAR PHASE – THE STAGE OF PREPARATION

Stage summary: Several eggs begin to develop, but only one of the eggs will fully mature and prepare to be released from the ovary.

Hormones involved: FSH and oestrogen.

- The first day of your period is considered to be day one of your cycle. If pregnancy has not occurred during the last cycle, the production of the hormone progesterone has already begun to decline. This drop tells your uterus to shed its lining, also called the endometrium, which is a soft tissue bed that grows every month in anticipation of receiving a fertilised egg. If an embryo has not implanted, the lining is no longer needed and is shed as a woman's period.

- Our body automatically starts preparing itself for the next cycle by sending signals to the hypothalamus and the pituitary gland in the brain. The pituitary secretes the hormone FSH, or follicle stimulating hormone, which promotes the growth of the ovarian follicles. At the end of this phase, only a single ovarian follicle containing an egg will reach maturity (usually!).

- The growing egg follicle secretes the hormone oestrogen, which dominates this phase of the cycle.

- Rising oestrogen levels start building up a new uterine lining all over again. It consists of special tissue containing mucus-producing membranes, glands and blood vessels, all of which are under the influence of oestrogen.

Day 13 to 16

OVULATORY PHASE – THE FERTILE PHASE

Stage summary: Ovulation takes place and the corpus luteum forms.

Hormones involved: Progesterone and LH.

- Once the follicle has matured and oestrogen levels are high enough, the body prepares for ovulation, or the release of the egg from the ovary. High oestrogen levels cause the pituitary gland to release a surge of luteinising hormone, or LH.
- The sudden increase or surge in the levels of the LH hormone can be used as a predictor of ovulation. The levels of this hormone can be measured at home by using specialised ovulation predictor kits.
- LH weakens the membrane of the ovarian follicle, enabling the mature egg to leave the ovary.
- The egg is released from the ovary, leaving behind an empty shell that forms the corpus luteum, a structure that produces the hormone progesterone.
- Ovulation can occur anytime between day 10 and day 17 of your cycle. This is considered to be the most fertile phase of your cycle.
- Under the dominance of progesterone, the endometrium starts to thicken, blood vessels develop further and glands start storing nutrients required for nourishing the fertilised ovum.

Day 16 to 28

LUTEAL PHASE – THE CONCLUSION STAGE

Stage summary: The matured egg is fertilised, resulting in pregnancy or, in the absence of fertilisation, the cycle ends in a regular menstrual period.

Hormones involved: Progesterone.

- If the mature egg meets a sperm cell, it may be fertilised and implanted in the uterus. The corpus luteum will continue producing larger amounts of progesterone to support the survival and growth of the fertilised ovum.
- Failure to conceive will cause the corpus luteum to degrade or break down. The drop in the levels of progesterone signal the shedding of the uterine lining formed earlier. This will be the start of the monthly menstrual flow.

The menstrual cycle in PCOS

PCOS can completely disrupt your normal menstrual cycle. Although irregularity of menstruation (oligomenorrhea) is the most commonly seen menstrual feature of PCOS, women may suffer from a spectrum of menstrual disturbances. These abnormalities can range from very heavy periods to the complete absence of menstruation. Some women suffer from too frequent (more than one period per month), scanty and incomplete periods, regular but heavy periods with profuse bleeding, or irregular periods (oligomenorrhea) with eight or fewer periods per year.

And if that wasn't confusing enough, some women may even experience normal and regular menstrual bleeding but without ovulation. In fact, anovulatory bleeding (bleeding without mid monthly ovulation) has been reported in up to 20% of women who report normal menstrual cycles.[35]

Winning back ovulation

Absence or irregularity of ovulation is a major roadblock between you and pregnancy. So, re-establishing regular ovulation is your first goal in the journey from infertility towards motherhood. Persistent efforts and commitment are two things you need to pack in your bag before you set off on this amazing journey.

Research strongly suggests the natural and lifestyle changes recommended in this book to be effective in improving fertility. However, some couples choose to skip this route and fast forward to the option of using infertility treatment. Although obscenely expensive, many couples consider this option to be their best shot at getting pregnant. While IVF treatments can help you conceive, your PCOS will continue to hold power over your body. The genes you pass on to your child will still be influenced by your health status, including obesity, Insulin Resistance and metabolic syndrome. These factors affect and adversely influence your child's health for his or her entire lifetime. If your child is a girl, she may be more likely to develop PCOS. Remember, her eggs are developing while she is *in utero.* What you do now can potentially affect the health of your grandchild!

> *"In the midst of winter, I finally learned that there was in me an invincible summer."*
>
> **Albert Camus**

IVF comes with the potentially life threatening risk of ovarian hyperstimulation syndrome, or OHSS, which is seen with the use of synthetic hormones for stimulating ovulation. Additionally, PCOS can also affect the outcomes of the IVF treatment. Some studies have shown that obese women with PCOS undergoing IVF had lower fertilisation rates, lower implantation (the process of the fertilised egg becoming embedded in the uterus) rates and higher miscarriage rates.[36] My intention is not to distress couples who want to try IVF, but I do want to encourage each and every one of you to naturally manage – and potentially overcome – your PCOS, possible anovulation and infertility. The plus is – you are not just fighting for your fertility, you are fighting for a long, healthy, happy life. A life that will give you the healthful years to watch your children grow up.

If you find that you still need medical assistance, your IVF (or other assisted fertility procedure) will be more likely to succeed.

As an important aside, a healthier mum means a healthier baby. You will also be in a far healthier position to enjoy your pregnancy and motherhood.

Let food be thy medicine

Hippocrates – the father of modern medicine – regarded food as the most powerful medicine. Food has an incredible ability to help you lose weight, boost ovulation, normalise your menstrual cycle and balance your hormones. Eating well and limiting foods that aren't good for you is a huge step towards health, and carrying a happy, healthy baby on to a safe delivery.

Check out this list of foods that will help in boosting your natural fertility:

Fish power: Oily fish like salmon, mahi-mahi, tuna, mackerel, and sardines are rich in omega-3

OMEGA-6 AND OMEGA-3 FATTY ACIDS

Studies have shown that women with PCOS have an imbalance of 'eicosanoids' – complex molecules derived from essential fatty acids like the omega-6 and omega-3 fatty acids.

Omega-3 fatty acids facilitate pregnancy in women suffering from infertility by improving blood flow to the uterus. Including healthy portions of oily fish and nuts that are rich in these fatty acids before and during pregnancy can help in reducing the risk of miscarriages, pregnancy induced hypertension, premature births and birth defects in babies.

http://www.cbn.com/health/naturalhealth/drsears_fertility.aspx

Women and Omega-3 Fatty Acids, *by Saldeen, Pia MD, PhD*; Saldeen, Tom MD, PhD, Obstetrical & Gynecological Survey, *October 2004, Volume 59 Issue 10, pp722-730.*

essential fatty acids. These fats help in reducing inflammation, boosting ovulation, improving insulin sensitivity and in lowering blood cholesterol levels. Due to the risk of mercury and lead contamination in fish, however, limit your intake of fish to less than 340 grams (12 ounces) per week.[37]

Go nuts: Nuts like almonds and walnuts are great sources of proteins, omega-3 fatty acids, B vitamins, vitamin E and fertility boosting minerals like copper, manganese, magnesium and potassium. The abundance of antioxidants in nuts puts them in the super food category. Walnuts and almonds contain precursors which naturally boost and balance our hormones and favour the maturation of eggs in the ovaries. In fact, walnuts were a symbol of fertility to the Romans.[38]

> *"The corpus luteum that produces the progesterone needed for sustaining the pregnancy is found to carry high levels of beta-carotene (i.e. vitamin A). Research studies show that cows that are deprived of beta-carotene developed ovarian cysts and suffered from poor ovulation. Their fellow mammals – we humans – can also suffer from similar effects if deprived of beta-carotene, aka vitamin A."*
>
> http://www.cbn.com/health/naturalhealth/drsears_fertility.aspx
>
> Making Babies: A Proven 3-Month Program for Maximum Fertility (Google eBook), by Sami S. David, Jill Blakeway, Hachette Digital Inc., 2009.

Fill up your plate with colours: Indulge in plenty of yellow, red, orange, green, blue and purple fruits and vegetables. The richer the colour, the greater the amount of phytonutrients in the fruits and vegetables. Bring variety to your food plan by including a variety of organic produce in a wide spectrum of colours. Orange fruits and vegetables contain vitamin A or beta-carotene; these are especially important nutrients for both male and female fertility. Vitamin A can balance hormones and even prevent early miscarriages.[39]

Phytoestrogens: Plant-based oestrogens are very helpful in balancing your hormones. They are most effective in the form of the isoflavones that are found in garlic, and legumes such as lentils and chickpeas. They help in correcting the oestrogen dominance of anovulation, and often found in women with PCOS. Isoflavones also boost the levels of SHBG (Sex Hormone Binding Globulin), which helps to reduce the amount of free testosterone and oestrogen in the blood.[40]

Whole grains: Gluten-free whole grains can be precious when it comes to improving fertility in women, as well as men. Examples of these grains include oats and brown rice.

Whole grains are rich in the vitamins and minerals that boost ovulation. The B vitamins and vitamin E in whole grains also help in improving the quality of the cervical mucus (mucus produced in the cervix of the uterus), which is vital for the safe entry of sperm into the uterus. Whole grains are rich in complex carbohydrates which may also help you to deal with Insulin Resistance and the other hormonal imbalances that come with it. They also contain plenty of folic acid, which is crucial for the proper growth and development of the baby and for preventing birth defects like spina bifida.

"As you can see, there are fantastic foods that have many nutrients packaged up inside. Eggs, nuts and seeds are the force for new life. As such, they contain the nutrients essential to create this new life. Imagine what that can do for you – and your fertility!"

Dr Rebecca Harwin

Lean proteins: Healthy protein is important for the health of both parents, and especially their eggs and sperm. Think fish, eggs, nuts, seeds and meat. Meat should be organic, free-range and unprocessed, with the fat trimmed. Avoid organ meat. Eat a palm-size portion of these healthy proteins two to three times each day.

Minerals: Oysters are well-known as an aphrodisiac. Maybe this is due to the abundance of the mineral zinc, which is known to boost fertility. Other foods containing zinc include nuts, duck, eggs, spinach and mushrooms.

Vitamins:

- Vitamin A, among other important functions, helps the little hairs inside the fallopian tubes gently move the egg towards the womb. Foods that are a good source of vitamin A include egg yolk, carrots, rockmelon, peaches, sweet potato and mango.
- The B vitamins are important in helping your baby reach an ideal weight, and they help support progesterone levels. If taking a supplement, take these B vitamins together (rather than separately). Foods to include are sesame and sunflower seeds, egg yolk, and sardines.
- Vitamin C helps us produce sex hormones, very important in maintaining a pregnancy. It has even been shown to help induce ovulation in anovulatory women. Most people know that oranges are rich in Vitamin C, but other citrus fruits, bananas, strawberries, cabbage and cauliflower all contain this important vitamin too.
- Vitamin D is important for your health, and the health of your growing baby. It is especially important for the growth of bones and teeth. We have become paranoid of the sun, but getting enough sunshine is important to your health. Staying in the sun until you are no more than slightly pink is enough to give you a rich supply of vitamin D. Time required depends on your skin colour and the time of year. Herring and egg yolks are good dietary sources of vitamin D.

Antioxidants: Oxidative stress causes toxic effects on the maturation of the potential egg (oocyte). Melatonin and vitamin E have been shown to decrease oxidative stress. One study found "melatonin is likely to improve oocyte quality and fertilisation rates".[41]

This is good news. Foods high in vitamin E include sesame seeds, olive oil, egg yolk, almonds, olives and sunflower seeds.

Other lifestyle changes

- Regular practice of exercise, Yoga, meditation and/or relaxation techniques will help you lose weight, balance your hormones and manage stress.
- Quitting anti-pregnancy habits like smoking, junk food, alcohol and caffeinated drinks will help both you and your partner significantly increase your chances of having a healthy pregnancy and a precious baby.
- Regular Chiropractic care will optimise the health of your nervous system (including your brain), and your biomechanics – prior to, during and after pregnancy. This is important for your health, and the health of your baby.

Paving the path for a healthy pregnancy

The famous saying 'an apple doesn't fall far from the tree' is so very true in women with PCOS. If the complex tangle of metabolic disturbances associated with PCOS is not improved before pregnancy, there is a chance your child will suffer the same health conditions – and complications – as you. Dr David Barker and his colleagues at the University of Southampton in England called this phenomena 'foetal programming'. This, and many similar studies, show that the mother's health status has a profound impact on the environment in the uterus, which in turn affects the growth and development of the baby. This effect is so strong that it programs the baby's organs for health or sickness from the time the baby is conceived.[42] In earlier chapters, we have seen how maternal PCOS can precipitate related changes in the ovaries of female babies right from the womb.

There is, however, a bright side to this sticky situation. In the same way your poor health can reflect negatively on your baby's health, positive changes in your lifestyle and food plan during the pre-conception period can be extremely beneficial for your baby-to-be. These modifications should be started well before you conceive and should be continued throughout pregnancy and breastfeeding. Then, as you teach your children healthy lifestyle choices as they grow, you will have a profoundly beneficial effect on not only them, but future generations. It is the responsibility of every parent to make positive changes to their lifestyle before they attempt to conceive a pregnancy to ensure a healthy baby and eventually, a healthy adult. By being as proactive as possible, you decrease your future child's risk of PCOS, obesity, diabetes, heart dis-ease, allergies and asthma to name but a few.

Pre-conception care for both parents is suggested for at least four months before trying to conceive. Here are a few things you need to do as a part of the pre-conception period:

1.   Lose weight: If you are not at a healthy weight, try to lose at least a few kilograms before you begin your attempts at conception. Weight loss has been consistently shown to boost fertility, and obesity during pregnancy is associated with a higher risk of pregnancy-induced diabetes and hypertension.

When you are trying to lose weight before conception, aim for a well-balanced food plan that includes a lot of nutritious foods. Also, rotate various groups of foods like gluten-free whole grains, fruits, vegetables, legumes, nuts, seeds, fish, lean organic meats, and poultry regularly through your meals.

Weight-loss diets are not, however, recommended during

pregnancy and breastfeeding as they can deprive both mum and baby of essential nutrients. Stay away from popular crash diet regimens that advise you to eat high amounts of unhealthy protein and few carbohydrates. Such extreme diets – which include more meat and little or no green vegetables – are not healthy for either yourself or your baby. Even back as far as 1953, it was observed low-fibre diets may be responsible for increased rates of eclampsia, stillbirth and neonatal deaths.[43] These diets can cause deficiencies in essential vitamins and minerals that are necessary for conception as well as a healthy pregnancy.

Weight loss during pregnancy has also been shown to stress the baby growing inside the womb.

2.   Detox your environment: Environmental pollutants like mercury, lead and other chemicals like PCBs, parabens and phthalates can all have hazardous effects on your fertility, conception, pregnancy and the precious baby that will grow in your womb. The first step in detoxification is to identify the toxins. Then purge your household and workplace of all harmful chemical cleaners,

> *"The only safe synthetic chemicals are the ones you are not exposed to!"*
>
> **Dr Samuel Epstein, Professor of Environmental and Occupational Medicine at the School of Public Health, University of Illinois Medical Center, Chicago.**

cosmetics, toiletries and so on. Every item that has a complicated list of chemical names listed on its label must go. Remember, there are no chemicals that can be called 'safe'.

Here are a few more points that you should keep in mind:

- Organic fruits, vegetables, meats, poultry and home care products will protect you and your family from exposure to harmful chemicals and toxins.
- Drinking filtered water that is not stored in plastic bottles is

best. Water should be filtered to remove fluoride, chloride, bacteria and other contaminants.

- Avoid eating processed, pre-cooked, refined and packaged food as much as you can. Eat fresh, home-cooked and well-balanced food.

- Use natural cosmetics and toiletries that do not contain any harmful chemicals. There are some great companies specialising in this area.

3.   Don't forget to detox your body: It is vitally important for you – and your partner – to detoxify your bodies. Your body may play host to many toxins – lodged in your skin, lungs, liver, gut and fatty tissue. Our body produces certain by-products during our metabolism that can stagnate in the body, leading to toxicity. In addition, your body must also fend off external toxins. It must protect us as much as possible. If we can't eliminate a toxin, we bind it within our cells. Our body is always trying to adapt and keep us safe. With the onslaught of modern day living, sometimes we actively need to give it a hand.

When speaking about detoxification, the two most important areas to focus on are the gut and the liver, in that order. Consider a possible oestrogen detox also. As we have discussed, many women with PCOS are oestrogen dominant. You are now well on your way to a healthier you, and a healthier baby. Don't forget to encourage your partner to come along with you on this detox journey. After all, his sperm are crucial to creating a healthy new life. I highly recommend you see a health care practitioner who specialises in detoxification for advice, support and appropriate supplementation.

NOTE: You and your partner should complete your detoxification at least four months prior to the remainder of your preconception period. It takes three months to produce a healthy egg, and four months to produce a healthy sperm.

NOTE: Never detox while pregnant – the toxins released may affect the baby growing in your womb.

Your gut: A correctly functioning gut is vitally important to a correctly functioning body. If you remember back to Chapter 5 ('Your Gut – Learn how to stop that embarrassing wind, relieve your bloatedness and tummy pain, and improve your PCOS'), you will know this is the perfect place to start. Any food you ingest or supplements you take will be more beneficial with a healthy gut. Your gut also influences the rest of your body, because toxins can be allowed into your body if your gut is permeable. To help your gut efficiently remove stagnant faecal matter, become less permeable, absorb nutrients more efficiently and provide a quality home for your helpful gut bugs, we need to include foods that are rich in natural fibre like gluten-free whole grains, legumes, fruits and vegetables. Also:

- Drink plenty of warm pure water to help flush out the toxins.
- Add pre and probiotics, supplemental glutamine (the putty filler for the holes in your gut) and omega-3s.
- Include aloe vera, honey and ginger.
- Remove offending foods and drinks. In this book, I have included information about foods that will sustain and improve your health, both long-term and for detoxification purposes. You will also find the foods you should remove from your food plan.
- Exercise, relaxation and yogic breathing (pranayama) also help in enhancing your body's natural detoxification processes.
- Reduce stress and eat consciously.

Your liver: A sluggish liver contributes to toxic build-up. Fatty liver – not uncommon in women with PCOS – will contribute to suboptimal liver performance. Below are some ways that will help you detoxify your liver:

- Ensure a steady supply of antioxidants like vitamin C, vitamin E and vitamin A in your food plan. Eat plenty of citrus fruits and include fresh red, yellow and green vegetables. Gluten-free whole grains, nuts, seeds and vegetable oils are great sources of vitamin E. These antioxidants help in removing the toxic chemicals stored in the fat cells and assist by making them water soluble. This, in turn, eases their excretion.[44]

- Liver cells also need natural sulfur containing amino acids like cysteine and taurine for an effective detox. Cruciferous vegetables like cabbage, cauliflower, broccoli, Brussels sprouts, raw garlic, onion, chives, leeks and shallots, all contain natural sulfur compounds that help the liver in detoxifying our body.[45]

- Add turmeric (curcumin) and green tea.

- Adding healthy protein, methylating vitamins such as the B vitamins and folic acid, minerals, antioxidants and relevant supplements is critical. As you detoxify, you need the right nutrients to assist in making this process a healthy and successful one.

- Soaking in an Epsom salts bath (a bath tub full of water, with hospital grade or U.S.P. grade Epsom salts or magnesium sulfate added) can help you to detox your liver and skin. Magnesium and sulfur, both of which can be absorbed via the skin, help the liver to purge the body of toxic chemicals. Use one to two cups of Epsom salts per tub full of water and soak for 15–20 minutes. You can enjoy this bath several times a week.

- Try dry body scrubbing, massage, and gentle movement/exercise.

- Drink enough pure water.
- Get enough rest.

Oestrogen detox: Removing excessive oestrogen is important on the journey to health for many women with PCOS. The detoxification steps we have already discussed are also very important now. If you remember back to Chapter 5 and the enzyme betaglucuronidase, you will appreciate the true importance of a gut detox for correcting oestrogen levels.

So:

- Ensure a high fibre food plan.
- Eat organic foods.
- Minimise pesticides and herbicides, and other xenoestrogens.
- Increase phytoestrogen intake, found in flaxseeds and sesame seeds.
- Avoid beef and chicken, unless the meat is organically grown, hormone-free and free-range.
- Add supporting supplements like indole-3-carbinol.

NOTE: I discuss detoxification in greater detail in my 12-week 'Conquer Your PCOS' home study course. You can find out more information by going to *www.ConquerYourPCOSCourse.com*

4.   Take your supplements: Make sure that you include whole foods and supplements that provide you with the necessary amounts of folic acid, iron, zinc, calcium and omega-3 fatty acids. These are extremely important for conception and the early development of your baby.[46]

5.   Avoid your vices: Alcohol, smoking, street drugs, refined sugars and caffeine are your worst enemies when trying to conceive. They are not just bad for your own health, but also hazardous for your unborn baby. Removing these habits right from the pre-conception period is important to ensure healthy conception and a healthy baby. This rule also applies to your partner. Being a man does not make him immune to their hazardous effects. Alcohol, smoking and other toxins affect the quality of sperm, all of which will decide the success of your attempts to get pregnant. I have included a special report on male fertility 'Crush Male Infertility – How to Put the Lead in his Pencil and Improve the Quality of his Lead' as a bonus for you to download and share with your partner. Go to *www. ConquerYourPCOSNaturally.com/BonusReports* to grab your FREE copy now.

6.   Drink enough pure water!

The best advice I can give you when you and your partner are ready to try conceiving is to wait. What, I hear you say. Wait? Yes, that's right! It really is worth

> *"Most people spend more time, consideration and money planning their annual holiday, than planning the creation of a brand new life!"*
>
> *Dr Rebecca Harwin*

spending the time, money and effort – for at least four months prior to trying to conceive – preparing, improving your health, detoxifying, de-stressing and ensuring adequate nutrition, all by following the steps above. Four months is not a long time when you consider the benefits to you, your partner, and the future of your children.

When you are ready, read on for more information on how to track your ovulation, optimising your fertile period for conception.

How to predict ovulation

The two most important things to know when you are looking to become pregnant are whether or not you are ovulating, and when. Initially, keeping track of ovulation lets you see where you are in regard to ovulation, and where you need to head.

When you are ovulating, you are in the most fertile zone in your cycle. This is important, as well-timed intercourse around this period is critical in achieving a successful and natural conception.

Ovulation is a silent process. Some women feel a slight twinge 'at the exact moment when the egg is released', known as 'mittelschmerz'. This is German for 'middle pain' and known in medical terms as 'ovulation pain' or 'midcycle pain'. The latest research shows it may take 15 minutes for ovulation to occur. Successful prediction of ovulation results when you can observe the changes in your body that come before and after ovulation.

Below are some methods you can use to accurately predict ovulation:

1.   Basal body temperature (BBT)

Your basal body temperature is your body temperature when you are completely at rest. This temperature is taken using a special basal body thermometer or fertility thermometer. Basal body temperature will start rising as ovulation occurs (as progesterone is produced) and will continue to rise until it reaches its highest point. The rise in basal body temperature is by up to 1 degree Fahrenheit (0.5 degree Celsius) during the time of ovulation. The three days or so during the mid-cycle, when this activity happens, will be your most fertile period.

Women are advised to take their basal body temperature starting from the first day of their cycle. The temperature is recorded in the morning by placing the thermometer under your tongue when you are still resting in bed, before any movement. Take this temperature at the same time every day, because a later hour means a higher temperature and can lead to inaccurate readings. To understand your pattern of ovulation and fertile days, you need to chart your BBT for three to four months.[47] For easier tracking, it is better to maintain a separate chart for each cycle. Your temperature needs to be recorded on a chart similar to the one given below. You can also track your cervical mucus (which we will discuss briefly). By comparing your BBT and cervical mucus, you can determine when, and if, you have ovulated. Go to *www.ConquerYourPCOSNaturally.com/Ovulation* to download your copy of the ovulation chart I use in practice. Here you will also find detailed charting instructions. These charts are a good guide for you, and are most helpful to a health care professional specialising in this area.

	MONTH 1			MONTH 2 (and so on)		
	DAY 1 (Date)	DAY 2 (Date)	DAY 3 ... to DAY 28	DAY 1 (Date)	DAY 2 (Date)	DAY 3 ... to DAY 28
BASAL BODY TEMPERATURE (BBT)						
CERVICAL MUCUS						

2.   Cervical mucus testing

Cervical mucus is the mucus normally produced at the mouth (cervix) of your uterus. This mucus can be a clear and wet, translucent and stretchy, or thick and flaky discharge from the vagina. The qualities of this mucus such as the colour, amount and consistency, will be affected by the hormonal changes that occur around ovulation. These changes will help you in predicting your ovulation. Cervical mucus testing is done by checking the mucus before urination by collecting it with toilet paper or between your thumb and forefinger from your vaginal opening. Make sure you wash your hands first. Check the cervical mucus for these factors:

- **Consistency:** Describe the consistency of the cervical mucus depending on its external sensation like dry, moist/damp, or wet. The wetter the sensation, the more fertile you are.
- **Amount:** The amount of cervical mucus will increase as you get closer to ovulation.
- **Texture:** The texture of the cervical mucus can vary from none or pasty in the non-fertile phases, to creamy or milky in the stages after ovulation, to clear, stretchy or like raw egg whites at ovulation. Each woman is different and mucus can also vary from cycle to cycle.

Just like the basal body temperatures, it is best to chart your cervical mucus qualities for three to four months to understand your ovulation pattern.

3.   Ovulation prediction kits (OPKs)

Your body experiences a surge in the hormone LH (refer to Chapter 3) just before ovulation, which will usually follow in the next 24–48 hours after this surge. These kits, which can be used at home, will help you assess your LH levels and in turn the most fertile days of your cycle.

Time it well

When you understand your own fertility rhythms using the above methods, you are in a better place to enhance your chances of conception. Remember, an egg is viable only for a period of 24 hours after ovulation. However, the most fertile period of your cycle spans up to a period of 5–6 days before ovulation and ends 24 hours after you have ovulated. After intercourse, the sperm can survive for up to five days inside your reproductive tract. This is the main reason behind this wider window in your fertile period. Making love during this fertile period significantly increases your chances of getting pregnant.[48]

Take a cue from your feelings

You need not to only rely on tests and charts, your own emotions and feelings are also indicative of ovulation. Research has shown that a woman's interest in flirting with their partner and in sexual intercourse increases just before ovulation (approximately five days before the surge in the levels of their LH hormone). Men are also found to be more protective and possessive of their partners during the most fertile phase of the woman's cycle.[49] So, alongside the temperature taking, chart plotting and mucus testing, be attentive to your own feelings and desires. Some studies have shown that women can conceive outside their fertility window as well.[50]

Oh, and don't make the process mechanical. You don't need to wait for your fertile period to enjoy each other, and connect. Relax, and remember you are creating new life with the one that you love. Be romantic, spontaneous, go away on a holiday, spend the day in bed, give each other massages and try new things. An orgasm helps a women conceive. Enjoy the practice!

Can't get enough?

Go to *www.ConquerYourPCOSNaturally.com/ BonusReports* to grab your FREE bonuses.

As an additional bonus, you'll also receive Dr Rebecca's *'Conquer Your PCOS'* monthly newsletter for FREE. You'll discover even more PCOS advice, easy-to-apply practical tips, PCOS-friendly recipes, and become a *'Conquer Your PCOS'* VIP.

Act now and join us and the 'Conquer Your PCOS' community!

Also, follow Dr Rebecca at:

www.Facebook.com/ConquerYourPCOS
and
http://Twitter.com/ConquerPCOS

Chapter Fourteen

Acne And Excessive Hair Growth

Tips and secrets for clear, smooth, radiant skin

"Hirsutism is a problem that is more than skin deep"

Dr Rebecca Harwin

Hirsutism is defined as the growth of dark terminal hair in women, located in areas we normally associate with men – the lip and chin, chest, down the centre of the abdomen, around the nipples and on the lower back.[1]

This condition should not be confused with the normally dark hair growth often seen in women of Mediterranean or Indian descent or those with naturally darker skin.[2] It is estimated that 60–80% of women with PCOS have some degree of hirsutism.[3] This excessive hair can be so embarrassing for some women that they would rather cover up and stay home than risk being exposed to the world.[4]

Hirsutism is caused by a combination of increased androgen production by the ovaries, a reduction in Sex Hormone Binding Globulin (SHBG) and an increase in 5-alpha reductase, an enzyme that activates androgens – particularly testosterone – in the hair follicles. The severity of hirsutism is also influenced by the hair follicles' sensitivity to androgen.[5]

In PCOS, the ovaries may overproduce androgens. Normally,

SHBG binds to excessive androgens, keeping them inactive until they are excreted in the urine. If the levels of SHBG are too low, free androgens, particularly testosterone, circulate in the blood. Once testosterone reaches the hair follicles, the enzyme 5-alpha-reductase activates the testosterone into dihydrotestosterone (DHT) and it causes the hair to become thicker and darker. DHT can also cause male pattern baldness in women.[6]

Acne – it's not just for teenagers

One of the most common skin disorders, acne is synonymous with the androgen excess of puberty and PCOS. It is estimated that up to 80% of women with moderate to severe acne have PCOS.[7] Acne consists of excess sebum (oil) production and bacteria in the pores. Blackheads and whiteheads arise from pores clogged with sebum, dead skin and bacteria. Many women with PCOS have acne on the face, chest, back and neck.[8]

The following grading system is used by doctors to define the severity of acne:

- **Mild:** Small, painless comedones (large white heads or black heads) and fluid filled acne (papules) less than 10 in number found mainly on the face.

- **Moderate:** Papules with redness about 10–40 in number and pus-filled acne (pustules) about 10–40 in number found mainly on the face.

- **Moderate to severe:** Numerous papules (40–100), pustules (40–100) with large comedones (40–100), affecting the face, upper chest and back, sometimes accompanied by larger node-like inflamed acne up to five in number.

- **Severe:** Inflamed and painful acne with nodes and cysts (fluid-filled lesions) found mainly on the chest and face along with many papules, pustules and comedones.[9]

How are hirsutism and acne alike?

The high levels of active testosterone that trigger dark, thick hair growth also cause the glands in the skin to produce more oil and exacerbate acne.[10]

Like hirsutism, excessive androgen levels are associated with the presence of acne, but the severity of the acne does not correlate with the amount of androgen excess. Some studies have shown that reduced SHBG, which contributes to increased levels of free testosterone, is associated with increased acne. In addition, hyperinsulinemia and Insulin Resistance contribute to androgen excess and worsen hirsutism and acne symptoms.[11]

Other causes of hirsutism and acne

The hirsutism and acne associated with PCOS do not appear overnight. They are a result of slow and gradual changes to your hormonal balance. If these conditions develop suddenly, they may be caused by:

- Tumour or cancer of the adrenal gland.
- Tumour or cancer of the ovary.
- Cushing's syndrome (a condition where the body produces abnormally high levels of the hormone cortisol).
- Certain medications like testosterone, danazol, anabolic steroids, glucocorticoids, cyclosporine, minoxidil, phenytoin, etc.[12]

Conventional treatments

Conventional treatments aim to reduce free testosterone by synthetic anti-androgen drugs, or the oral contraceptive pill or, more recently, by decreasing insulin levels with insulin-sensitising drugs. Widely used to treat the hyperandrogenism and Insulin Resistance of PCOS, some scientific researchers question their efficacy as well as their safety.[13] The side effects of these treatments may carry risks that are, often times, more severe than the initial condition. Cosmetic therapies including waxing, tweezing, laser hair removal, photofacials, laser skin resurfacing, chemical peels and dermabrasion may help remove excessive hair and acne, but they do not address the underlying cause of excessive androgens levels.

Food as therapy for hirsutism and acne

Food plan and lifestyle changes, including losing weight where needed, and exercising, are key to rebalancing your hormones, improving your PCOS, and reducing hirsutism and acne, but they take time.[14] These changes are the safest and most long-lasting way to reduce excess hair, male-pattern balding and acne. They also address the body as a whole.

Several research studies have shown how an appropriate food plan can help rebalance hormones. One study reported that women who stayed on a low calorie diet for at least six months lost weight and reduced Insulin Resistance. Their levels of SHBG increased, which reduced the amount of free testosterone in their blood. As expected, the women reported a reduction in the severity of their hirsutism and acne symptoms.[15]

Another study treated young men with severe acne for 12 weeks with a diet containing 25% protein and 45% low glycaemic foods. At the end of the 12 weeks, the men had lowered Insulin Resistance and less acne.[16] Yet another study reported that a vegetarian diet that included a high percentage of plant proteins resulted in decreased free testosterone and DHEA in the blood.[17]

An Italian study showed substituting meats, eggs and dairy products with fruits, vegetables, whole grains and legumes significantly reduced excessive testosterone levels. These changes also increased SHBG.[18]

These studies support eating more protein, less carbohydrates and adding low glycaemic load foods to reduce Insulin Resistance and decrease testosterone production. Low glycaemic load foods are those that do not cause a significant or sudden blood sugar rise. One note of caution when selecting foods – *low calorie* is not the same as *low glycaemic* and vice versa. Here are some tips for selecting healthy, low glycaemic load foods:

- Fruits and vegetables are low glycaemic and low calorie foods. Increasing your daily servings of fruits and vegetables will not only help you balance your hormones but will also give you the additional nutritional benefits such as vitamins, minerals, fibre and antioxidants, to help you heal your skin. Apples, strawberries, blueberries, cherries, raspberries, grapefruit, oranges, peaches and kiwi fruit are some of the best choices. Artichokes, asparagus, broccoli, cauliflower, celery, cucumber, eggplant, carrots, yams, green beans, leafy greens (lettuce, spinach, kale, chard, mustard greens), summer squash and tomatoes also meet the low calorie and low glycaemic load standards.

- Gluten-free whole grains, peas, beans and lentils are low on glycaemic load and calories. They contain complex carbohydrates, dietary fibre and the nutrients required to help balance your hormones.

- Foods that contain harmful types of saturated fats, white flour, sugar, artificial colours or flavours, and preservatives are not part of a healthy food plan. These ingredients wreak havoc on hormonal balance and weight management, making the symptoms of PCOS, including excess hair and acne, worse. Processed foods such as lunch meats and boxed dinners contain many of these unhealthy ingredients and should be avoided.

Other treatments for hirsutism and acne

Changing your food plan, and weight loss where needed, reduce the 'male' hormones responsible for acne and hirsutism. What else can help you overcome these embarrassing complaints?

- Licorice root (glycyrrhiza) has been shown to be effective in decreasing testosterone levels.[19]
- Fish oils help reduce inflammation, which may be of benefit in acne.
- Zinc aids in healing and so may be helpful for acne.
- Reducing or eliminating alcohol helps to decrease the levels of 'male' hormone in your blood.
- Stress management.
- Detoxification can help to balance your hormones, improve your health and your skin.
- A natural topical antibacterial skin lotion may help reduce acne.

Can't get enough?

Go to *www.ConquerYourPCOSNaturally.com/ BonusReports* to grab your FREE bonuses.

As an additional bonus, you'll also receive Dr Rebecca's *'Conquer Your PCOS'* monthly newsletter for FREE. You'll discover even more PCOS advice, easy-to-apply practical tips, PCOS-friendly recipes, and become a *'Conquer Your PCOS'* VIP.

Act now and join us and the 'Conquer Your PCOS' community!

Also, follow Dr Rebecca at:

www.Facebook.com/ConquerYourPCOS
and
http://Twitter.com/ConquerPCOS

Chapter Fifteen

What If I Don't Make Changes?

*What PCOS will do to you if you
don't take steps to conquer it now*

You've received a diagnosis of PCOS, and there are so many questions to get answers to. Those questions may include: "What other problems am I at risk of?" and maybe even "What else can go wrong?..."

These are important questions because there are real health problems in addition to the potential difficulties in getting pregnant and giving birth, maintaining a healthy weight, irregular periods, facial hair and acne. Women with PCOS have an increased risk of diabetes, metabolic syndrome, sleep issues (including sleep apnoea), cardiovascular dis-ease, mood disorders and certain types of cancer.[1,2,3,4] We'll go through these one at a time, giving conventional approaches as well as alternative approaches. We'll discuss nutritional and lifestyle advice, as well as herbs and supplements that may help. Always remember to talk to your suitably qualified health care professional. Work with them – and have them work with you – in order to achieve optimal and vibrant health.

Getting pregnant and giving birth

The irregular cycles and the hormonal imbalances in PCOS can make getting pregnant difficult. And, depending on whether you are on medication for PCOS or any of the complications, when you *do* get pregnant, those medications may have to be discontinued.

Many physicians use a combination of metformin (Glucophage) and clomiphene (Clomid, Serophene) to induce ovulation.[5,6,7] Clomiphene induces ovulation but has some serious possible adverse effects including multiple pregnancy, blood clots and problems with vision.[8] Metformin, often used to increase the body's sensitivity to insulin, is also used to treat the hirsutism and menstrual irregularities associated with PCOS. The use of metformin is controversial[9] – in the US, it is not FDA-approved for the treatment of PCOS.[10] Metformin can cause an upset stomach, an increase in lactic acid and an increase in the levels of homocysteine – which is considered a marker for cardiovascular dis-ease risk. Clomiphene should *not* be used in pregnancy because it may cause birth defects.[11,12] In addition, it's important to know that if you are on metformin, this medication depletes the essential B vitamins, folic acid and B12.[13,14]

One of the best – though not necessarily the simplest – ways to increase your chances of getting pregnant is to lose weight, where needed.[15,16,17] Weight loss can restore ovulation and fertility – and also results in decreased serum levels of testosterone and an improvement in the insulin profile, blood glucose levels and an increase in the amount of Sex Hormone Binding Globulin (SHBG) – all good news.[18,19,20,21] In one study, of women who lost 2–6% of their body weight – nine out of the 15 women began ovulating regularly.[22] In another study, the average weight loss was 6.8 kilograms – nearly *all* the women began ovulating and almost half of the women became pregnant within six months. The risk of miscarriage was decreased as well. (There was a less than 20% rate of miscarriage after the weight loss. This was in the same group of women had experienced a 75% rate of miscarriage before they lost the weight.)[23]

Reducing calories (but not having a very low calorie intake) and increasing exercise, has been shown to be an important aspect of weight loss, rather than any specific diet – like low protein, high protein, low fat or high fat.[24,25,26] One study examined the Atkins, Ornish, Weight Watchers and Zone diets – they all seemed to produce the same results as far as weight loss[27], so the main goal should be to use a lowered calorie diet that *you* can stick with.

It's *very* important to find a way to lose weight that you can maintain. One of the best ways – and with a high success rate – is to eat foods with a low glycaemic index.[28] You can do this by increasing the amounts of vegetables in your food plan, eating only complex carbohydrates (gluten-free whole grain breads, legumes, vegetables), limiting the amounts of animal fat and avoiding processed or refined foods. The idea is to eat the same sorts of foods your grandparents and great-grandparents ate – and they didn't eat TV dinners, instant rice, canned peas or processed bread – they ate lots of vegetables, fruits, whole grains, beans, lentils and drank pure water. They also consumed less red meat – and ate more fish. It is *very* important to lose weight with healthy, whole foods because then, you not only *lose* weight, but you tend also to keep the weight off. Plus, the healthier your food plan, the healthier – and happier – *you* will be. Organic foods are even better because they reduce the number of environmental toxins you are exposed to – and these toxins can worsen inflammation and hormonal imbalance in your body.[29] (For more information on how inflammation works and how to decrease it, see Chapter 7 'Oxidative Stress – What is it, why it can kill you, and how to defeat this fertility assassin'.) Whole food diets are what humans evolved eating. Your body will simply work better for you when you choose a whole food, food plan. *Whole foods* are *unprocessed foods* – which means they take longer to digest... *that* means you don't get as hungry as you do when eating processed foods... and *that* means you are much more likely to eat less.

Eating healthy is great, but it is also very important to increase your activity and exercise level. Keep it simple and easy at first. Start with short walks and increase the lengths of your walks slowly but steadily. It can help to have a specific goal with your walk – you can walk to your friend's house, take your dog (or cat!) for a walk, walk to the shopping centre instead of driving and even walk to the grocery store... if you have to carry groceries back, you can even get a head start on burning off the calories from your dinner. Exercise doesn't have to mean running a marathon. You can increase your physical activity by walking up or down stairs rather than taking the elevator or escalator. You can make two trips to the filing cabinet instead of one; you can park further away from your home or office. Start an activity you will enjoy – like gardening, visiting a park or zoo, bird watching or, if you are fortunate enough to live by the ocean, seashell collecting. The point is to find something you enjoy that involves moving. If it is something you enjoy, you are more likely to keep on doing it.

Increased risk of diabetes

Woman with PCOS are at risk of developing diabetes – this has been recognised for some time.[30] As mentioned, many physicians will treat women with metformin, often considered to be the 'first-line' treatment for the hirsutism, fertility issues, Insulin Resistance, weight reduction and the irregular periods associated with PCOS. Metformin may, or may not, decrease the risk of developing diabetes. There have been few studies proving metformin decreases the risk of diabetes.[31] One study (a meta-analysis) did find that treatment with metformin reduced the risk of diabetes by 40%.[32] On the other hand, it has been shown that losing 5–10% of total body weight can restore ovulation, improve insulin sensitivity *and* reduce the risk of diabetes.[33] While no one is suggesting that weight loss is easy, it is possible. The steps throughout this book will help you here. Weight loss has other advantages as well. Think about it – there are no negative effects of healthy weight loss. Compare this to the potential side effects of metformin. These side effects include diarrhoea, nausea, vomiting, abdominal bloating, possible vitamin B12 deficiency (that can result in anaemia, stomach and gastrointestinal problems and neurological problems) and possible lactic acidosis (where your body becomes much more acidic than it should be because of a build-up of lactic acid).[34] Given the fact that as little as 5–10% weight loss can improve your health so much and reduce your risk of diabetes, isn't it at least worth considering?

Another aspect of a whole food, food plan should be mentioned here. A whole food diet includes the complex carbohydrates you get from fruit, vegetables, whole grains, beans and legumes. Complex carbohydrates take longer to digest, and this means that your blood sugar levels remain more stable. Stability of blood sugar reduces the risk of diabetes.[35,36]

Increased risk of metabolic syndrome (MS) and cardiovascular dis-ease

Metabolic syndrome is also known as syndrome X, cardio-metabolic syndrome, and Insulin Resistance syndrome. Metabolic syndrome is defined[37] as a central obesity with a combination of two of the following treated or untreated conditions:

- Increased triglycerides
- Decreased HDL (often referred to as 'good' cholesterol)
- Blood pressure greater than 130/85
- Increased fasting blood sugar levels.

'Central obesity' means the weight around your midsection and is defined differently for different ethnic groups.

Thirty-three to 40% of women with PCOS who are overweight have metabolic syndrome, or MS. About 37% of young girls with PCOS have metabolic syndrome as well.[38] The general agreement among researchers is that the excess weight is what puts women at risk for both PCOS and MS.[39]

Cardiovascular dis-ease can include problems with blood pressure, atherosclerosis (sometimes called hardening of the arteries), increased cholesterol and an increased risk of strokes. But... guess what... your food plan plays a very important role in cardiovascular dis-ease.[40] And – the same dietary suggestions made throughout this book will also help reduce your cardiovascular dis-ease risk.

Losing weight will decrease your risk of metabolic syndrome as well. Just so this doesn't begin to sound like an echo chamber, the risk of metabolic syndrome can be decreased not only by good, whole food nutrition, but also by herbs and supplements. You can even incorporate some herbs and spices into your food to make them more interesting to eat. For example, cinnamon has been shown in a number of studies to balance blood sugar levels.[41,42,43] Triglycerides and total cholesterol were also reduced. Other herbs such as fenugreek, gymnema and prickly pear have shown promise in this area.[44]

Other supplements to think about are the antioxidants. (See Chapter 7 'Oxidative Stress – What is it, why it can kill you, and how to defeat this fertility assassin' for a full explanation on antioxidants and what they can do for you). Examples of great antioxidants include vitamins B2 (riboflavin), C and E, fish oils, CoQ10, resveratrol and alpha-lipoic acid. Other helpful antioxidants include grape seed, bilberry, turmeric (curcumin), thyme, ginkgo, milk thistle and green tea. Don't forget – many herbs can be added to your meals – thyme and curcumin (the basis of curry sauces) can be used in many meals. You can drink green tea... and, fruits and berries are chock-full of antioxidants, so go ahead and have a bunch of blueberries, strawberries, cranberries, currants or grapes. Choosing organic produce is helpful. Remember that the skins of these fruits and berries contain lots of fibre as well as being full of antioxidants. Fibre is a great way to help maintain steady blood sugar levels and maintain overall gut health.

Sleep issues and sleep apnoea

Sleep apnoea is defined as episodes during sleep when a person stops breathing for a short period of time. This leads to loss of sleep and an increased level of stress. Stress in this case means not only that overwhelmed, tired and exhausted feeling, but also an increase in substances such as cortisol.[45,46] Over time, these chemical changes can cause serious and lasting damage. Sleep apnoea is associated with being overweight.[47] It is also affected by hormones. All the reproductive hormones, including oestrogen, progesterone and testosterone, play an important role in getting to sleep and staying asleep – and, play an important role in sleep apnoea.[48] Low progesterone, common in patients with PCOS, has been recognised as being correlated with poor sleep.[49,50] And, the fact is if you are tired or exhausted because of night after night of disturbed sleep – well, nothing else seems to go well either. Again, weight loss can definitely help. A number of people benefit from using the CPAP masks, which help to maintain a regular breathing rhythm while you sleep.[51,52] Another approach which has worked well in helping women around the time of their change to menopause (perimenopause) to sleep, is supplementing with progesterone.[53] Women in perimenopause, and women with PCOS, can have low progesterone levels. Talk to your health care professional about natural, short-term progesterone replacement.

These are the natural progest*erones* and not the synthetic progest*ins*. They can be used as a cream or gel, or in oral forms. The natural progesterones are used also to treat irregular cycles. Progesterone can be used on a temporary basis very safely[54] until you feel better and/or you regain regular ovulation patterns. For some women, progesterone supplementation can be a godsend. When you can't sleep well, it can be difficult to have a positive outlook and be able to embark on the food plan and lifestyle suggestions given here. It is worth addressing any sleep issues at the same time you begin a weight loss program – after all, sleep deficiency is itself a risk factor for weight gain[55,56] and Insulin Resistance.

The increased risk of cancer

Women diagnosed with PCOS appear to have a higher risk of certain types of cancer, including cancer of the colon, kidney, the endometrium, ovaries, breast (in postmenopausal women) and oesophagus.[57,58] There is some evidence that the risk for uterine cancer may be the same as in women without PCOS[59], and that there may not be an increased risk of breast cancer[60], but overall, it is generally recognised that women with PCOS have higher rates of uterine, ovarian and breast cancer.[61] It is thought that the higher levels of oestrogens combined with the lower levels of progesterone, common in women with PCOS, increases the risk of cancers associated with organs that are hormone dependent – like the uterus, the ovaries and the breast.

Many physicians believe that using oral contraceptives in PCOS – mainly to 'restore' the menstrual cycle, reduces the risk of endometrial and uterine cancer.[62] The conventional wisdom is to use contraceptives containing nonandrogenic progestins such as norgestimate and desogestrel.[63] Part of the problem here is that irregular periods are not the *cause* of PCOS – they are a symptom. Simply causing a monthly bleed does not regulate the menstrual cycle. It also does not address the more basic underlying problems of weight, Insulin Resistance, too much testosterone and oestrogen, and insufficient levels of progesterone – it's a Band-Aid covering a more serious problem. We know that while Band-Aids are useful at times, they are best used for superficial problems, not deeper ones.

Another concern is the dependence on synthetic hormones – we know there are risks associated with these.[64,65] We simply don't know what, specifically, causes most cancers. We do know by strengthening the body and minimising the risks – by removing toxicity and deficiency to attain purity and sufficiency – by minimising exposure to environmental and food toxins, and the toxins in our personal and household care products, by eating healthy, whole foods, by reducing stress and improving the way we think, and by losing weight when needed (overweight and obesity are independently associated with a greater risk of cancer[66]), we can significantly reduce, or even eliminate, our chance of developing cancer. Once again, you can minimise the risk of cancer by losing weight, thereby better controlling Insulin Resistance, decreasing the amount of testosterone in your system and re-balancing the oestrogen and progesterone.[67] Another additional approach is to address the underlying inflammation in being overweight. Having additional weight causes a body-wide inflammatory process.[68,69,70,71,72] To reduce this inflammation, there is a lot you can do. Eat anti-inflammatory organic foods such as vegetables, fruits, nuts and seeds, and fish. Drink pure water and green tea. You can use anti-inflammatory herbs and spices in your cooking or as supplements – these include basil, cayenne pepper, thyme, turmeric, garlic, onions, rosemary, parsley, oregano and cinnamon – that's quite a variety in taste. The good news is that an anti-inflammatory food plan is the same food plan required for a low glycaemic weight loss program...

This all helps you to lose weight, feel better *and* diminish your risk of cancer.

Mood disorders and PCOS

There is evidence that women and girls diagnosed with PCOS have greater rates of depression and anxiety.[73,74,75,76] These conditions may not even have been noticed or diagnosed. If you are feeling anxious and/or depressed, please talk to a counsellor or therapist about how you are feeling. These problems can lead to a vicious cycle, as depression and anxiety can also decrease fertility and affect your weight.[77] Depression and anxiety can develop because of self-image issues, fertility problems, loneliness, pre-menstrual syndrome (PMS), pre-menstrual dysphoric disorder (PMDD), and fear for the future and overall quality of life concerns.[78,79] These seem to be mainly centred around the hirsutism, weight and acne problems associated with PCOS.[80,81] The good news is that most of the symptoms of depression and anxiety can be improved and resolved with counselling, support (such as that found in PCOS support groups), weight loss where needed, exercise, sunshine and the restoration of healthy sleep patterns.[82] Vitamins like B6, minerals like zinc, and fats like omega-3 can be very useful in improving emotional and mental challenges. The more your health improves, the better you will feel mentally and emotionally. The more balanced your hormones, the more balanced your mind.

Summary

PCOS is a complex condition which places women at risk for a number of other conditions. By empowering yourself and making changes to improve your overall health, you also significantly reduce your risk of suffering further health challenges.

Can't get enough?

Go to *www.ConquerYourPCOSNaturally.com/BonusReports* to grab your FREE bonuses.

As an additional bonus, you'll also receive Dr Rebecca's *'Conquer Your PCOS'* monthly newsletter for FREE. You'll discover even more PCOS advice, easy-to-apply practical tips, PCOS-friendly recipes, and become a *'Conquer Your PCOS'* VIP.

Act now and join us and the 'Conquer Your PCOS' community!

Also, follow Dr Rebecca at:

www.Facebook.com/ConquerYourPCOS and *http://Twitter.com/ConquerPCOS*

Chapter Sixteen

Communicate Well

A guide for your loved ones to understand and support you

> *"The single biggest problem in communication*
> *is the illusion that it has taken place"*
>
> *George Bernard Shaw*

One of our greatest responsibilities is to offer unconditional support to our partner and our loved ones. Whether the woman you love has just been diagnosed with Poly Cystic Ovary Syndrome, or it has been a part of her life for a long time, you will be her teammate in facing and managing this condition on a day-to-day basis. Many women living with PCOS find themselves facing much more than just the physical effects of this syndrome. PCOS changes her body, and leaves many women feeling de-feminised and unattractive. This can make it challenging to achieve and maintain feelings of confidence in a relationship. If she is a family member or a friend, your support is also crucial if she is to overcome PCOS. In this case, where I refer to her 'partner', I am also referring to other loved ones.

Understanding what PCOS is

To find out more about PCOS, go to Chapter 1 'What Is PCOS? Plus, where to start'.

If your partner has been living with PCOS for a long time, there's a good chance that both of you already know a good deal about it. If she has just been diagnosed, or has recently opened up to you about her condition, then you have a lot to learn. PCOS affects every woman differently and the key to understanding what your loved one is facing lies not only in knowing what her symptoms are, but in knowing what causes them. This book is a great resource. Take the time to read it and educate yourself about what causes PCOS and the ways in which it can affect the body. Keep it handy as a reference. When you and your partner need information, or a way forward, refer to it.

Consulting with a PCOS specialist is helpful. Someone who specialises in PCOS can provide valuable, focused information and insight that other practitioners may not be able to offer. If your partner doesn't already have one, seek out a local specialist who is knowledgeable about natural and alternate treatments, as opposed to one who uses pharmaceutical drug therapy. Strengthening her body, and bringing it back into balance, should always be your focus. If you cannot locate a local specialist, consider making a trip to meet with one on occasion. Consult with a Nutritionist or Naturopath who will be able to offer advice tailored to your partner's needs. Accompany her to see the specialist whenever possible. Play an active role during the appointments. Remember that, if you do not have PCOS and do not experience the symptoms for yourself, educating yourself about PCOS is vital to understand what your partner is going through.

While you can collect books, consult with appropriate specialists, and gather the right information, your prime source of information will most likely be your partner. She may or may not know all the scientific details, but she lives with PCOS every day.

Understanding what PCOS is to your partner

While she is part of a group of women who share the common reality of living with Poly Cystic Ovary Syndrome, your partner is also an individual who lives with changes and thoughts unique to her. Understanding what living with PCOS means for her will help you be more supportive on a daily basis, and when she is feeling particularly challenged by her symptoms.

When was she diagnosed? Has PCOS been a part of your partner's life for years, or is it something she is just discovering?

A recently diagnosed woman is likely to be faced suddenly with all sorts of feelings and questions, starting with what exactly PCOS is, why she has it, and what she needs to do from now on. She may feel distraught over discovering that she has a syndrome which can affect her hormones and her body so dramatically, or she may feel relief at finally having an answer. Much of the information available – and there is not a lot in mainstream channels – is incomplete or simply inaccurate.

Someone who has been living with PCOS for years will have been through the initial challenges, and hopefully has made some major adjustments to her lifestyle. However, she may feel hopeless after years of unsuccessfully trying to find a way forward.

What are her unique symptoms? There are tell-tale signs and symptoms of PCOS, such as increased 'male' hormone, causing acne, excessive hair growth or male pattern balding, through to obesity and/or absent periods. Some women with PCOS have more severe health challenges than others, while other women experience milder symptoms. What you can see, however, may not be the same as what she feels. For more detailed information about the various PCOS symptoms, please see Chapter 3 'Restore Your Hormonal Balance – Discover what your hormones do, and the secrets to balancing them once more', which covers the hormonal imbalance in PCOS and the resulting symptoms.

Know what symptoms your partner has, how severe they are for her, and how long she has lived with them. She has probably been living with the symptoms since before she was diagnosed and her symptoms may have developed or changed over time. Know exactly which ones she deals with, and how they make her feel.

What challenges has she faced? Find out what specific challenges she must handle. Does she experience a lot of physically painful symptoms? Does she struggle with her weight? Is she uncomfortable with her body? Know what challenges she has faced in the past, know what challenges she faces in the present and know that new challenges may arise in the future. If you define those challenges you need to overcome together, you can find a way forward as a couple. You will also have ideas on the specific challenges that need to be addressed.

How has she managed PCOS thus far? Some women have made many positive changes in their lives after being diagnosed, but a great percentage – in my clinical experience and from the emails I receive – have been unable to find the right answers to manage their PCOS well. Have her tell you what she does, what she knows works and what doesn't. Know if she has specific eating habits, a specific workout routine, if she relies heavily on pharmacotherapy (get access to the special bonus report 'Could the medications you've been prescribed for your PCOS be aggravating, or even con-tributing to, your condition?' at *www.ConquerYourPCOSNaturally. com/BonusReports*) and how many lifestyle changes she has made in order to conquer her PCOS. If she still faces challenges, or if PCOS is new for her, then now is a good time for both of you to come up with a plan for managing, and eventually conquering, her Poly Cystic Ovary Syndrome together.

Is it time for a change? No matter how long PCOS has been part of your partner's life, now is as good a time as any to evaluate – or re-evaluate – her approach to it. Educate and re-educate yourselves as necessary. Examine what point she is at, define any challenges, examine your approaches and decide together what needs to change.

Understanding what PCOS means for your relationship

As with any relationship, you and your partner should work as a team and commit to facing your challenges together. This includes facing PCOS. Life throws us all sorts of challenges, and PCOS will come with challenges of its own. Be prepared – and dedicated – to work things through. Take on an active role in the management of your partner's PCOS – beyond awareness of the disorder, visits to healthcare professionals and decision-making. If you are willing to make changes to your own lifestyle, it could make a big difference in how successfully she commits to managing her condition. Making these changes together will also solidify your partnership. You may be surprised at how beneficial some changes are to your own health.

Understand what she needs

Everyone has different needs and expectations from their partner. You should discuss and be aware of what your partner needs, specifically, to help her on her journey. Living with any chronic health challenge can be an alienating or isolating experience. Whether you are male or female, let your partner know that she is not alone. Express, and show her, your support. Make a genuine effort to understand her needs.

Emotional support

PCOS causes hormonal imbalances which can affect her emotions. Being supportive through the emotionally challenging periods can help ease the stress associated with these times. Offering emotional support while she's facing a challenging period is important. Let her know that you are there for her, and that you want to help her work through her feelings. Women with PCOS are more likely to suffer from depression, anxiety and low self-esteem. Due to the upsetting nature of some of the signs and symptoms, she may also not be upfront about how she is feeling. She may know she is feeling irrational, but at the same time be unable – or too embarrassed – to express the reasons for her emotional state. Be patient.

TIP: Do not invalidate her feelings, or assume if she is upset, it must just be her 'PCOS talking'.

Encouragement and motivation

Making lifestyle changes can be difficult for anyone. Making the lifelong lifestyle changes vital to the maintenance of good health and overcoming PCOS can be extremely daunting. *Your* motivation and encouragement are often just as important as *her* dedication to maintaining healthy habits.

Be encouraging on a day-to-day basis – encourage her to take the steps to improve her health and overcome her PCOS – no matter what hardships she is facing.

Nutritional needs

This book is jam-packed full of nutritional advice and tips – including the right foods needed to overcome PCOS. Regardless of the severity of her PCOS, speaking with a nutritional specialist (i.e. a Naturopath, or a Nutritionist) and improving her food plan is *essential* in overcoming PCOS. Be aware of which foods to avoid, and which foods are beneficial. Stock the pantry and refrigerator accordingly.

Nutrition plays a huge role in conquering PCOS. There are ideas and suggestions on what to eat – and what to eliminate from your food plan – provided throughout this book. Chapter 17 'Eat your way to health – The best food plan to conquer your PCOS' will consolidate this information for you. You can grab a copy of my recipe book 'Conquer Your PCOS – 50+ Delicious and Healthy Recipes For Optimal Living' from *www.ConquerYourPCOSNaturally.com/RecipeBooks.* This recipe book is full of PCOS-friendly breakfast, lunch, dinner and snack ideas.

Communicate

Communication is the key in all relationships, and communicating about your partner's PCOS regularly is important. You may not always be able to recognise how she's feeling. Ask her, and ask her to let you know when she needs to talk. You do not want PCOS to become the focus of your lives together, but be aware when she's experiencing any challenges. Discuss how you both feel about the changes being implemented to improve her PCOS – and your lives. If she thinks that it's time to try a new approach, then hear her out, decide together on a way forward, and take action accordingly.

Eat together

Your partner is at greater risk for obesity, diabetes and heart dis-ease than women living without PCOS. Both of you need to eat the right foods, in the correct proportions for your weights, activity levels and individual nutritional needs. This is one very important area where a collaborative effort will make a huge difference in overcoming her PCOS, and achieving real health for both of you. The ideal food plan for your partner is also the ideal food plan for you. If you both implement and enjoy the foods recommended in this book, you will keep each other on track and both improve your health.

Certain foods can be extremely detrimental to your partner's health, especially in excess, so prevent temptation by keeping those foods out of the house, and encourage each other to eat healthy portions. Find some healthy alternatives to your favourite treats that the two of you can enjoy. Do not encourage her to starve herself. A very low calorie diet is damaging to artery walls. Plus, if she does not receive the nutrients needed, she will not improve her health, lose weight, or overcome her PCOS. Eating five smaller meals daily (breakfast, lunch, dinner and two snacks) helps keep her body in balance, her energy levels stable and contributes to a good mood.

Exercise together

Physical activity has a huge impact on health. Movement – or lack thereof – also affects how your partner's PCOS manifests. Incorporating additional activity can really improve her quality of life. Contributing to overall well-being, decreased cravings, improved insulin sensitivity, balanced bathroom scales and reduced depression, are just some benefits to a more active life. When you exercise as a team, you will both benefit. When one of you doesn't feel like exercising, the other can be the motivating partner. You will both feel better once you introduce additional physical activity in to your lifestyle.

Exercise will help to control obesity, and obesity and PCOS often go hand-in-hand.

Cardiovascular exercise strengthens the heart, which is extremely beneficial to a woman with PCOS.

Strength training is something many women approach with caution, but it really is a valuable addition to the fitness program of a woman with PCOS. Strength training does not need to have the same effect as body-building. Lean muscle burns fat, which helps fight obesity even when not exercising. As with cardio, start with low weights and work your way up as you become stronger.

Remember to warm up, cool down and stretch every session. Stretching regularly will help your body to recover from exercise and improve your overall well-being. Also remember that exercising doesn't have to take place in a gym. Consider all the activities that you both enjoy, and any incidental activity you can incorporate, and you might be surprised at how active your lifestyle can become.

If neither one of you is accustomed to exercising, start at a level you are comfortable with and slowly build to more strenuous routines.

Support each other – regardless of what level each of you is at – and encourage each other to improve. As your fitness improves, push yourself. If you do not feel comfortable exercising without the guidance of a professional, or you want to get greater results, seek out a personal trainer. Be sure that you discuss your current fitness levels and where you can safely start. You may need to be under your physician's care. See Chapter 11 'The Magic of Movement – How to simply and easily incorporate movement into your life. Plus, I reveal the single training tip for quicker, easier fat loss and hormonal control' for more information about movement. Or for specific exercises, and greater detail and advice, grab yourself a copy of my 12 part 'Conquering Your PCOS' home study course at *www.ConquerYourPCOSCourse.com*

Be a team

You are who you hang out with. Pursuing a healthy lifestyle together is about more than just mutual support. People influence each other, and we have a tendency to become more like the people we spend time with. If you and your partner are committed to one another, each of your being healthy will encourage and motivate the other to do the same. Eating well and exercising together gives you both a common goal to strive towards. You'll be helping yourselves just as much as you'll be helping each other. This is a great opportunity to turn a health challenge into something positive.

Know what you both want

Children: The ability to conceive is a serious concern for many women who live with PCOS – whether through natural or assisted means. Irregular, or absent, menstruation and ovulation often occurs as a result of the hormonal imbalances common in this syndrome. If you both are ready for a family and are having trouble conceiving, there are a number of options available. Losing weight – where needed – tends to drastically improve a woman's ability to conceive. Maintaining a healthy lifestyle, addressing stress and consuming 'the right foods' are great for improving fertility. If, after trying everything else, you need to use assisted fertility techniques, the advantage is the changes you both have made together will improve the chances of these techniques succeeding. Remember also, it takes two to tango. Do not assume as your partner has PCOS, your fertility as a couple is all about her. If you are a heterosexual couple, read the bonus special report 'Crush Male Infertility – How To Put The Lead In His Pencil And Improve The Quality Of His Lead' by visiting *www.ConquerYourPCOSNaturally.com/BonusReports*. This report comes FREE with this book.

The lifestyle changes suggested throughout this book will improve your fertility as a couple, by improving the chances of becoming pregnant, and maintaining a healthy pregnancy through to term.

The future

Facing Poly Cystic Ovary Syndrome with your partner begins with adjusting your lifestyle together. Some environments are more conducive to maintaining an ideal lifestyle than others. Keep this in mind as you and your partner plan your future. Set several short-term goals to get your lives moving down the right track. Seeing these through will allow the adjustments you make to your life together to become sustainable lifestyle choices. Think about what you want in your future together, and determine what it will take to ensure that the two of you achieve your goals together.

Remember that you are a team, and that your relationship is a two-way street. As a woman living with PCOS, your partner will have several unique needs. She may rely on you to either provide direct help, or to support her through this process. Let yourself be empowered by the support that you provide her and let your unity enrich your relationship.

Can't get enough?

Go to *www.ConquerYourPCOSNaturally.com/BonusReports* to grab your FREE bonuses.

As an additional bonus, you'll also receive Dr Rebecca's *'Conquer Your PCOS'* monthly newsletter for FREE. You'll discover even more PCOS advice, easy-to-apply practical tips, PCOS-friendly recipes, and become a *'Conquer Your PCOS'* VIP.

Act now and join us and the 'Conquer Your PCOS' community!

Also, follow Dr Rebecca at:

www.Facebook.com/ConquerYourPCOS
and
http://Twitter.com/ConquerPCOS

Chapter Seventeen

Eat Your Way To Health

The best food plan to conquer your PCOS

"Let thy food be thy medicine and thy medicine be thy food."

Hippocrates, (460–377 BC)

Choosing the right food is critical for you in conquering your PCOS. We have discussed much about foods throughout this book. In this chapter, we will discuss which foods are great for you, and which are not. Plus, some simple tips to speed up your progress. Remember, there is so much more to the food you eat than simply trying to control your weight.

An ideal food plan for a woman with PCOS will include all the essential nutrients in terms of macromolecules, vitamins, minerals, cofactors, enzymes, fibre and vital energy. It will address deficiency and toxicity, balance your hormones, curb your cravings, encourage a feeling of fullness, and maintain an optimal body weight. The great news for your family is, this is the type of food plan they should also enjoy to bring them optimal health.

Important dos and don'ts

What to do:

1. Eat smaller, frequent meals.

2. Include lots of fresh vegetables and fruits.

3. Replace simple carbohydrates with complex carbohydrates.

4. Buy and eat organic food whenever possible.

5. Have a low glycaemic load (GL) food plan.

6. Include a great deal of salad. Eating salad at the start of your meal will help you feel full, increase the amount of nutrients you eat, and they taste great too.

7. Eat meals comprising protein, carbohydrates and healthy fat as this helps reduce Insulin Resistance.

8. Have 20–50 grams of fibre each day to fight Insulin Resistance. Sources include unsweetened coconut, flaxseeds, chia seeds, broccoli, cauliflower, celery, gluten-free whole grains, apples and dark leafy greens.

9. Include protein – eggs, nuts, fish and, less frequently, lean organic poultry and meat.

10. Use extra virgin cold pressed olive oil for cooking; flax oil, coconut oil or extra virgin cold pressed olive oil for salads. Add some apple cider vinegar, balsamic vinegar or lemon juice for extra taste.

11. Take the required supplements daily.

> ## SMALLER, FREQUENT MEALS DO HELP
>
> *Altering when and how often you eat can be helpful. Eat more frequently throughout the day, having four to six smaller meals instead of three large meals. This will contribute to you feeling full, and keep your blood sugar levels balanced. As a result, you are less likely to experience cravings and hunger pangs, averting you from grabbing that quick – often unhealthy – bite.*

12. If eating grains, choose gluten-free whole grains.

13. Add herbs and spices like curcumin (turmeric) and cinnamon to your food plan.

14. Add non-starchy vegetables, either raw or steamed.

15. Develop the habit of reading labels on food products you purchase.

16. Include plant sterols. For those with an imbalance in their cholesterol levels (dyslipidemia), plant sterols can help balance these levels.

17. Drink a minimum of two litres of pure water daily.

What not to do:

1. Never skip meals.

2. Avoid refined/simple carbohydrates.

3. Reduce, or remove, unhealthy fat.

4. Don't avoid healthy fats.

5. Avoid artificial sweeteners in all forms.

6. Limit consumption of alcohol.

7. Avoid high GI foods, such as refined bread, pasta and white rice.

8. Avoid a low fat, high carbohydrate diet.

9. Avoid fried foods.

10. Avoid non-organic animal products and fats.

Research you should know about:

Cinnamon helps in the prevention of insulin resistance and improves glucose and lipid profiles.[1]

A low carbohydrate, high protein diet helps Insulin Resistance. A high carbohydrate, low protein diet makes Insulin Resistance worse.[2]

A diet containing 25% carbohydrates improved Insulin Resistance, whereas a diet that included 45% carbohydrates did not.[3]

A small piece of dark chocolate once a week may help prevent heart dis-ease. Plus, the actual smell of chocolate, and eating a small amount, may even help you lose weight. If you want chocolate, buy good quality, dark chocolate.

If you are having cravings, a 15-minute walk will decrease, or overcome, your cravings.

42.5 grams (1.5 ounces) of nuts consumed everyday can lower the risk of heart dis-ease.[4]

Although not high in sugar, dairy does cause an increase in insulin secretion.

THE TIME YOU EAT

Does the time you eat make any difference?

Maybe, says Nutritionist Linda Morgan.

Blood glucose remained higher if the same meal was eaten at night, as opposed to the morning. Traditionally, we ate a big breakfast, moderate lunch, and small tea. It appears we may be well advised to take note of this.

There appears to be a body clock rhythm to insulin levels.

Recommended vegetables:

Alfalfa sprouts	Cauliflower	Mushrooms
Artichokes	Celery	Okra
Asian greens	Chard	Olives
Asparagus	Coleslaw, dry	Onions
Baby spinach	Cucumber	Radicchio
Bamboo spouts	Eggplant	Radish
Bean sprouts	Endive	Rocket
Bok choy	Fennel	Sea vegetables

Broccoli	Green beans	Snow peas
Broccolini	Kale	Spinach
Brussels sprouts	Kohlrabi	Sprouts
Cabbage	Leeks	
Capsicum	Lettuce – all types	

Other vegetables to include (if you are wishing to lose weight, limit to a total of one handful daily):

Carrots	Parsnip	Pumpkin
Corn	Peas	

Recommended fruits (if you are wishing to lose weight, one handful of these fruits can replace one handful of vegetables daily):

Apples	Grapefruit	Peaches
Apricots	Lemons	Pears
Avocado	Limes	Raspberries
Blackberries	Mulberries	Rockmelon
Blueberries	Nectarines	Strawberries
Cherries	Passionfruit	Watermelon

Recommended protein:

Chicken	Lamb	Scallops
Duck	Mussels	Squid
Eggs	Oysters	Tofu/Tempeh
Fish	Pork	Turkey
Kangaroo	Prawns	Veal

+ The above tables are courtesy of www.Metagenics.com.au

For suitable recipe ideas, go to *www.ConquerYourPCOS Naturally.com/OtherBooks*

Can't get enough?

Go to *www.ConquerYourPCOSNaturally.com/ BonusReports* to grab your FREE bonuses.

As an additional bonus, you'll also receive Dr Rebecca's *'Conquer Your PCOS'* monthly newsletter for FREE. You'll discover even more PCOS advice, easy-to-apply practical tips, PCOS-friendly recipes, and become a *'Conquer Your PCOS'* VIP.

Act now and join us and the 'Conquer Your PCOS' community!

Also, follow Dr Rebecca at:

www.Facebook.com/ConquerYourPCOS
and
http://Twitter.com/ConquerPCOS

Chapter Eighteen

Living In Wellness

The quest for an optimally well life, from PCOS to freedom

> *"Every person has the right to optimal health and vitality.*
> *To do this one simply needs to attain purity and sufficiency.*
> *You are worth it!"*
>
> Dr Rebecca Harwin

As our world, and our habits, have become more intricate, and we have moved further and further away from the life we are designed for, we have become sicker and sicker. This trend is continuing. As you have learnt throughout this book, the vast majority of sickness is not due to faulty genes. It is not due to your body lacking any particular drug. Your body is miraculous. Your body is constantly trying to find balance. If you give your body all that it requires, and remove any toxins, you will be well. This is also the key to conquering your PCOS.

I also need to address society's reliance of medication, particularly as it relates to PCOS.

Many women with PCOS are prescribed endless medications depending on their circumstance – the birth control pill, insulin sensitisers, anti-androgenic preparations, blood pressure tablets, cholesterol lowering medication, heart dis-ease and cancer drugs... But no-one seems to ask about the benefit/s to the person taking these medications, or about both the short-term or long-term outcomes associated with this form of treatment.

PCOS is often driven by Insulin Resistance, yet one of the most common medications used to 'treat' it – the pill – is known to cause Insulin Resistance![1,2]

As a Chiropractor, I took an oath to 'First, do no harm.' I take this oath seriously, as should all other health care professionals and companies.

Many people look to substances outside their bodies to regain health. In truth, this is a flawed concept, one that will never succeed. We search for more complex ways to become pregnant. We introduce toxic drugs into our bodies in the hopes of attaining health. Let me ask you a question.

If you had a wilting plant, would your first thought not be to give it water? Then sunshine? Then nutrients? Then remove toxins? If your pet dog vomited, would you first not wonder what he had eaten? You are no different. Yet, many people believe that to attain health, we need something other than the basics. If it is natural, wholesome, simple, in line with how we were designed, they think this can't be effective. The exciting facts are, research paper after research paper, shows *lifestyle measures* are the *best* option. Period.

How do you think you were designed? Do you really believe in your heart you are ill because of a lack of medication? Or are you ill, infertile, and not optimally vibrant and well because of your lifestyle choices and your environment? I can tell you with utmost certainty; science is showing us again and again the *basics* are what we need for a healthy life. Not drugs.

The most effective 'therapy' for type 2 diabetes is lifestyle choice. It been proven to be more effective than polypharmacy (i.e. the many drugs patients are given for one condition. For diabetes this is often one for cholesterol, one for blood pressure, one for insulin sensitising and so on). This should be of significant interest to you, given that women with PCOS have been found to have Insulin Resistance at the same level as those with diabetes.

The most effective 'therapy' for heart dis-ease is lifestyle choice. In the lifestyle heart trial[3], Dr Dean Ornish et al divided cardiac patients into two groups. The control group experienced a worsening in their condition. The group that engaged in lifestyle changes experienced not only a halting of their condition, but a reversal. They started getting better!

Research also shows lifestyle change is crucial in fighting cancer.

We know that lifestyle is the best medicine for chronic conditions. My question to you is do you really want to wait until you are diagnosed with cancer, heart dis-ease or diabetes before you decide to change your lifestyle? It is more powerful to act, and do so now. If you have already been diagnosed with PCOS, your body is crying out for a different lifestyle. You already have what could be considered a chronic health challenge. Move to implement change.

Your focus should be on what it takes for you to be optimally well. This is the very same thing it takes to conquer your PCOS. Focus on well-being, on optimal function. Do not simply focus on a symptom, or believe that being symptom-free, by default, equals health. Did you know for many people the first symptom of heart dis-ease is a fatal heart attack? Or that once ovarian cancer is detected, it is often late in its progression? Medicine defines prevention as regular check-ups for 'disease markers'. The interesting part of this is, by the time these markers indicate dis-ease, the 'disease' is already in progress. This is not *prevention,* this is simply *early detection.* Would you cover up the flashing light on your car dashboard telling you that you are almost out of fuel? Or would you fill the car before it conks out? If you are driving a Ferrari, would you put cheap fuel in the tank? Or would you only fuel your luxury vehicle with premium quality fuel? You are infinitely more important than any car!

The 'best medicine' for health is a great lifestyle. As Dr James Chestnut says, you need to eat well, move well and think well to be well.

"We spend our youth chasing wealth and our age chasing health."
Author unknown

Unfortunately, in western society, we often don't feel we can afford the cost of eating healthily and exercising regularly. With fast food stores offering food – and I say 'food' very loosely – at ridiculously low prices, many people find this cheap option appealing and easy. Interestingly, we often then spend our money on other things such as cigarettes, alcohol, movies, hobbies, daily coffee and the like. This is not prioritising health. Later in life when literally faced with 'spend or die', prioritising health becomes a necessity. Do you really want to have a life of suboptimal function culminating in an early death or worse, years of incapacitation? At this stage, the governments of many countries step in to pay for the expensive treatment medically recommended. Or, the effected individual then uses their accumulated wealth to try to regain the health they themselves lost over the years. As the story goes, is it better to put a fence at the top of the cliff, or an ambulance down in the valley?

For your sake and the sake of your family – or future family – please pay more attention, time and money to your health than you do to your car, annual holiday, plasma screen television or hobby. The effort will repay you one hundred fold. It's that simple.

Yours in wellness,

Dr Rebecca Harwin

Dr Rebecca Harwin
PCOS Expert, International Author, Chiropractor, Nutritionist

www.ConquerYourPCOSNaturally.com

Appendix One

Bonuses For Readers

BONUS 1:

Crush male infertility – How to put the lead in his pencil and improve the quality of the lead

Value: $37

Infertility is devastating. You burst into tears at your niece's first birthday, or feel a strong tug at the heartstrings when you hear a baby giggle, and wonder why it hasn't happened for you... If you and your partner have not yet been able to create your own little bundle of joy, you need this special report.

Many women blame themselves for not being able to conceive, but male infertility is an equal problem. In this bonus special report, I discuss the basics such as what sperm are, through to why male infertility is skyrocketing and what you both can do to turn this distressing situation around.

Included are:

- How to defeat the seven key sperm killers to make a healthy baby.
- The two critical nutrients required for his sperm to swim longer and straighter (absolutely necessary for them to reach – and fertilise – your egg).
- A common, inexpensive and readily available ingredient to

'unstick' his stuck together sperm and get them swimming freely again.

- The number one reason for his sperm to be damaged, resulting in infertility, DNA damage and increased rates of miscarriage, plus how to reverse this damage naturally.

A healthy sperm means more than just possible conception. It improves your chances of safely delivering a healthy, bouncing baby. This book discusses your health and your fertility. This report empowers him to improve his fertility too.

Go to *www.ConquerYourPCOSNaturally.com/BonusReports* now to grab this bonus special report for FREE.

BONUS 2:

What if the foods already in your cupboard could help you conquer your PCOS?

Value: $29

How would you know?

The nutrients in your food are critical to your well-being and to conquering your PCOS. But, which foods contain what nutrients?

This bonus list spells out what foods are rich in which nutrients. Simply look up the nutrient you are interested in, and below you will find a list of foods high in that nutrient. Easy!

Head to *www.ConquerYourPCOSNaturally.com/BonusReports* now to grab your FREE copy.

BONUS 3:

Could the medications you've been prescribed for your PCOS be aggravating, or even contributing, to your condition?

Value: $12

Do you really know what the medications you are being prescribed are doing to you? This bonus report tells you candidly why medication is not the answer to conquering your PCOS, and even worse than this – why it could be aggravating, or contributing to, your PCOS. This report contains the secrets the pharmaceutical companies don't want you to know!

You MUST read this free report now. Download it from *www. ConquerYourPCOSNaturally.com/BonusReports*

BONUS 4:

The First THREE modules of my home study course. This is an unbelievable bonus!

Value: $249

'Conquer Your PCOS' – The 12 Week Action Plan has been designed as a blueprint to guide you from where you are to where you want to be. I cover all the major PCOS health challenges and concerns, and more – in detail. I more or less hold your hand, touching base with you each and every day. There is NO OTHER COURSE like this available. This really is your chance to 'Conquer Your PCOS' once and for all. And you receive the first three parts for FREE, as my way of rewarding you for being an action taker and purchasing this book. Don't forget to go to *www.ConquerYourPCOSNaturally.com/BonusReports* to get a hold of this incredible bonus. If you want to see what exactly is included in this life-changing course, see below or go to *www. ConquerYourPCOSCourse.com*

Appendix Two

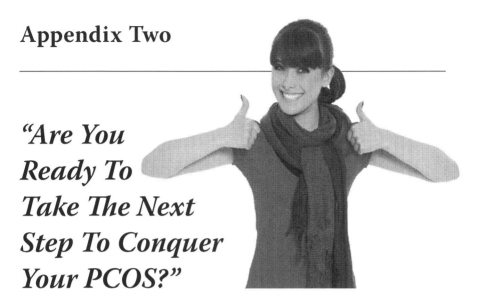

"Are You Ready To Take The Next Step To Conquer Your PCOS?"

You've now read the book and have an important foundation, and a way forward. But, imagine the benefits of more advanced secrets and strategies! The kind of information you won't find in your health professional's office. I've met women who've seen specialist after specialist, had test after test, and tried expensive remedies, procedures, even surgeries, without luck. If you want to short cut your journey to success, I have exciting news...

In **'Conquer Your PCOS' – The 12 Week Action Plan** you'll find a step-by-step, easy to follow, success blueprint. This course is designed to help you *turn your life around.*

Stop Struggling Now!

You'll receive:

Part 1: Secure THREE additional tools to help settle your wayward hormones.

Part 2: Learn easy, quick ways to help settle wind, bloatedness and gut pain.

Part 3: You'll get delicious and healthy recipes, to help ease great foods into your new food plan.

Part 4: Discover the vital keys to detoxifying safely to improve your health, fertility and weight loss. *PLUS:* Luxurious detox surprises to help you enjoy the process.

Part 5: Tips to transform your body. Reaching your ideal weight is more than simply reducing your food. We go through the next level of factors that influence your size.

Part 6: Learn even more about movement. *GIFT:* Many women with PCOS experience back pain, and this can seriously affect your ability to move and improve your health. Receive your copy of the 130 page eBook 'Conquering Your Back Pain'. You'll discover specifically what the research shows works, exercises to strengthen weak muscles and stretch tight muscles easily in your home, tips on posture and more.

Part 7: Learn further strategies for removing toxins from your environment and body. *GIFT:* Receive a pocket-size carry card with a list of the dangerous chemical codes, plus the affects these have on your health. I introduce you to companies that can make your life, and this transition, much easier.

Part 8: Breakthrough! Discover the next level of fertility facts. *VITAL TOOL:* Complete ovulation chart with instructions.

Part 9: Stress Quiz: Take this quiz to see if stress is playing a role in your health, and if so, just how much of a toll it is taking on your well-being. *PLUS:* 'The Secret Sleep Report'.

Part 10: Learn the secrets of relaxation.

Part 11: Take on your unsightly spots and embarrassing excessive hair and win. *GIFT:* Special Report – 'Seven Key Steps To Conquering Your Acne Naturally'.

Part 12: Acquire the skills and secrets to not only Conquer Your PCOS but to live a healthy, happy and long life.

BONUSES:

When you act now, for a limited time only, you'll receive 4 additional bonuses valued at $287! Go to *www.ConquerYour PCOSCourse.com* now to find out more information before I decide to take these bonuses down for good.

Bonus One: A quick and easy meditation audio to help you gain the upper hand over your stress. Simply download on to your MP3 player, burn to a CD, or listen straight from your computer.

Bonus Two: 'Conquer Your PCOS – 50+ delicious & healthy recipes for optimal living'. My recipe book – designed specifically for women with PCOS. Full of PCOS-friendly recipes for breakfast, lunch and dinner, as well as for a special occasion.

Bonus Three: Need more personalised professional guidance? *Save 25%* off your initial consultation with me when you invest in your copy of the 'Conquer Your PCOS' 12 part home study course.

Bonus Four: A bonus audio with EVERY module. Each audio focuses on a PCOS relevant topic to give you all the information to create the life you want.

Bonus Five: And much, much more…

To grab your copy of **'Conquer Your PCOS' – The 12 Week Action Plan,** with the above bonuses, additional weekly articles to guide you to success, plus daily tips, thoughts and advice, and other secret surprises along the way, head to *www.ConquerYourPCOSCourse.com* now and follow the instructions. This course will help you *turn your life around,* keep you on track, and provide the blueprint to guide you towards **Conquering Your PCOS.**

Win a personalised, one-on-one consultation with Dr Rebecca Harwin

You've finished 'Conquer Your PCOS Naturally'. Congratulations!

As you have started on the path to your new life, I want to give you the opportunity to jump forward in leaps and bounds.

For your chance to win, simply go to:

www.ConquerYourPCOSNaturally.com/Feedback

and complete the quick questionnaire.

Good luck!

References

CHAPTER 1 REFERENCES

1. Balen Adam H, Laven Joop SE, Dewailly Seang-Lin Tan Didier, 'Ultrasound assessment of the polycystic ovaries: International consensus definitions', Human Reproduction, Update Vol 9, Issue 6; 2003, p505-514

2. Carmina Enrico, Azziz Ricardo, 'Diagnosis, phenotype and prevalence of Polycystic Ovary syndrome', Fertility and Sterility, Vol 86, Supplement 1, July 2006, s7-s8

3. Azziz Ricardo, Dunaif Andrea, Ehrmann David, 'Polycystic Ovarian Syndrome (patient information page from the Hormone Foundation)', The Journal of Clinical Endocrinology & Metabolism, Vol 89, No 9, September 2004

4. Kelly Chris CJ, Lyall Helen, Petrie John R, Gould Gwyn W, Connell John MC, Sattar Naveed, 'Low Grade Chronic Inflammation in Women with Poly Cystic Ovarian Syndrome'. The Journal of Clinical Endocrinology & Metabolism Vol 86, No 6; 2001, p2453-p2455

5. Kuzelmeric Kadir, Alkan Nevriye, Pirimoglu Meltem, Orhan Una, Turan Cem, 'Chronic Inflammation and elevated homocysteine levels are associated with increased body mass index in women with polycystic ovarian syndrome', Gynecological Endocrinology, Vol 23, No 9; 2007, p505-p510

CHAPTER 2 REFERENCES

1. Tattersall Ian, DeSalle Rob, Wynne Patricia J, Bones, 'Brains and DNA: The Human Genome and Human Evolution', Bunker Hill Publishing Inc, 2007, p22

2. Reilly Philip, 'The strongest boy in the world: how genetic information is reshaping our lives', CSHL Press, 2006, p161

3. Griffiths Anthony JF, Wessler Susan R, Lewontin Richard C, Carrol Sean B, 'Introduction to genetic analysis', Macmillan, 2008, p471

4. http://www.cancer.gov/cancertopics/understandingcancer/geneticbackground/allpages/print

5. http://www.genetichealth.com/G101_Genetics_Demystified.shtml

6. Roof Judith, 'The Poetics of DNA' (Google eBook), U of Minnesota Press, 2007, p149

7. Komaroff Anthony L, 'Harvard Medical School Family Health Guide', Harvard Medical School, Simon and Schuster, 2004, p128

8. Griffiths Anthony JF, 'Modern Genetic Analysis: Integrating Genes and Genomes', Volume 2, Macmillan, 2002, p11

9. Church Dawson, 'The Genie in Your Genes' (Google eBook), Elite Books, 2009, p32

10. Lipton Bruce H, PhD, 'Nature, Nurture and Human Development', Journal of Prenatal and Perinatal Psychology and Health, 16(2), Winter 2001, p167–p180

11. Berger Kathleen Stassen, 'The Developing Person Through Childhood', Macmillan, 2005, p53

12. Sadava David, Heller H Craig, Hillis David M, Berenbaum May, 'Life: The Science of Biology', Macmillan, 2009, p356

13. Pelengaris Stella, Khan Michael, 'The Molecular Biology of Cancer', Wiley-Blackwell, 2006, p329

14. Roth Stephen M, 'Genetics Primer for Exercise Science and Health' (Google eBook), Human Kinetics, 2007, p73

15. Roth Stephen M, 'Genetics Primer for Exercise Science and Health' (Google eBook), Human Kinetics, 2007, p73

16. Chiras Daniel D, 'Human Biology', Jones & Bartlett Learning, 2010, p369

17. Farid Nadir R, Diamanti-Kandarakis Evanthia, 'Diagnosis and Management of Polycystic Ovary Syndrome', (Google eBook), Springer, Japan, 2009, p83

18. Nicholas L, Rattanatray L, McLaughlin S, Ozanne S, Muhlhausler B, Kleeman D, Walker S, Morrison J, McMillen C, 'Maternal Overnutrition and Undernutrition in the Periconceptional Period Results in Altered Expression of Hepatic Metabolic Genes in the Postnatal Lamb', Sansom Institute, Univ SA, Adelaide, SA, Australia

19. Hornstra Gerard, Uauy Ricardo, Yang Xiaoguang, 'The Impact of Maternal Nutrition on the Offspring', Karger Publishers, 2005, p7

20. Dolinoy Dana C, 'The Agouti Mouse Model: an Epigenetic Biosensor for the Nutritional and Environmental Alterations on the Foetal Epigenome', International Life Sciences Institute, 2008

21. Farid Nadir R, Diamanti-Kandarakis Evanthia, 'Diagnosis and Management of Polycystic Ovary Syndrome', (Google eBook), Springer, Japan, 2009, p97

22. Altchek Albert, Deligdisch Liane, 'Pediatric, Adolescent and Young Adult Gynaecology', John Wiley & Sons, 2009, p326

23. Church Dawson, 'The Genie in Your Genes' (Google eBook), Elite Books, 2009, p32

CHAPTER 3 REFERENCES

1. Challam Jack, 'ABCs of Hormones', McGraw-Hill Professional, 1999, p12

2. Rosdahl Caroline Bunker, Kowalski Mary T, 'Textbook of Basic Nursing', Lippincott Williams & Wilkins, 2007, P208

3. Farid Nadir R, Diamanti-Kandarakis Evanthia, 'Diagnosis and Management of Poly Cystic Ovary Syndrome', (Google eBook), Springer, 2009, p35

4. Diamanti-Kandarakis Evanthia, Nestler John E, 'Insulin Resistance and Poly Cystic Ovarian Syndrome: Pathogenesis, Evaluation and Treatment', (Google eBook), Humana Press, 2007, p146

5. Roush Karen, 'What Nurses Know ... PCOS', Demos Medical Publishing, 2010, p13

6. Blank SK, 'The Origins and Sequelae of Abnormal Neuroendocrine Function in Poly Cystic Ovary Syndrome', Human Reproduction Update, 2006; 12(4), p351-p361

7. Livingstone Callum, Collison Mary, 'Sex steroids and insulin resistance', Clinical science, 102, 2002, p151-p166

8. Holte J, 'Poly Cystic Ovary Syndrome and Insulin Resistance: Thrifty Genes Struggling with Over-Feeding and Sedentary Life Style?', Journal of Endocrinological Investigation, 1998, Vol 21, No 9 (114 p) (101 ref), p589-p601

9. Diamanti-Kandarakis Evanthia, Nestler John E, 'Insulin Resistance and Poly Cystic Ovarian Syndrome: Pathogenesis, Evaluation and Treatment', (Google eBook), Humana Press, 2007, p148

10. De Fronzo R, et al. 'Insulin Resistance: A Multifaceted syndrome responsible for NIDDM, obesity, hypertension, dyslipidemia and artherosclerotic cardiovascular disease', Diabetes Care, 14, 1991, p173-p194

11. Soliman PT, Wu D, Tortolero-Luna G, Schmeler KM, Slomovitz BM, Bray MS, Gershenson DM, Lu KH, 'Association between adiponectin, insulin resistance, and endometrial cancer', Cancer, 1;106(11), June 2006, p2376-p2381

12. Huber-Buchholz MM, Carey DGP, Norman RJ, 'Restoration of Reproductive Potential by Lifestyle Modification in Obese Polycystic Ovary Syndrome: Role of Insulin Sensitivity and Luteinizing Hormone', The Journal of Clinical Endocrinology & Metabolism, Vol. 84, No. 4; 1999, p1470-p1474

13. Sadock Benjamin J, Kaplan Harold I, Sadock Virginia A, 'Synopsis of Psychiatry: Behavioural Sciences/Clinical Psychiatry', Lippincott Williams & Wilkins, 2007, p123

14. Rao, 'Textbook of Gynaecology', Elsevier, India, 2008, p34

15. Nestler John E, Jakubowicz Daniela J, Falcon de Vargas Aida, Brik Carlos, Quintero Nitza, Medina Francisco, 'Insulin Stimulates Testosterone Biosynthesis by Human Thecal Cells from Women with Polycystic Ovary Syndrome by Activating Its Own Receptor and Using Inositol Glycan Mediators as the Signal Transduction System', The Journal of Clinical Endocrinology & Metabolism, Vol 83, No 6, 1998, p2001-p2005

16. Pasquali Renato, Casimirri Francesco, 'The impact of obesity on hyperandrogenism and polycystic ovary syndrome in premenopausal women', Clinical Endocrinology, Vol 39, Issue 1; July 1993, p1–p16

17. Weiner Cindy L, Primeau Margaret, Ehrmann David A, 'Androgens and Mood Dysfunction in Women: Comparison of Women With Polycystic Ovarian Syndrome to Healthy Controls', Psychosomatic Medicine, 66, 2004, p356-p62

18. Berrino Franco, Bellati Cristina, Secreto Giorgio, Camerini Edgarda, Pala Valeria, Panico Salvatore, Allegro Giovanni, Kaaks Rudolf, 'Reducing Bioavailable Sex Hormones through a Comprehensive Change in Diet: the Diet and Androgens (DIANA) Randomized Trial', Cancer Epidemiol Biomarkers Prev, January 2001, p10, p25

19. Nestler John E, Jakubowicz Daniela J, Falcon de Vargas Aida, Brik Carlos, Quintero Nitza, Medina Francisco, 'Insulin Stimulates Testosterone Biosynthesis by Human Thecal Cells from Women with Poly Cystic Ovary Syndrome by Activating Its Own Receptor and Using Inositol Glycan Mediators as the Signal Transduction System', The Journal of Clinical Endocrinology & Metabolism, Vol 83, No 6, 1998, p2001-p2005

20. http://www.labtestsonline.org/understanding/analytes/testosterone/faq.html#4

21. Norman Anthony W, Litwack Gerald, 'Hormones' (Google eBook), Academic Press, 1997, p348

22. Hemat RAS, 'Andropathy', Urotext, 2007, p350

23. Lavin Norman, 'Manual of Endocrinology and Metabolism', Lippincott Williams & Wilkins, 2009, p303

24. Balen Adam H, 'Poly Cystic Ovary Syndrome: a Guide to Clinical Management', (Google eBook), Taylor & Francis, 2005, p102

25. Azziz Ricardo, Nestler John E, Dewailly Didier, 'Androgen Excess Disorders in Women: Poly Cystic Ovary Syndrome and Other Disorders', (Google eBook), Humana Press, 2006, p248

26. Longcope C, Feldman HA, McKinlay JB, Araujo AB, 'Diet and Sex Hormone-Binding Globulin', The Journal of Clinical Endocrinology & Metabolism, Vol 85, No 1, 2000, p293-p296

27. Michaels Jillian, van Aalst Mariska, Darwin Christine, 'Master Your Metabolism: The 3 Diet Secrets to Naturally Balancing Your Hormones for a Hot and Healthy Body!' (Google eBook), Random House Inc, 2009, p42

28. Behl Christian, 'Diet and Sex Hormone-Binding Globulin, Estrogen, mystery drug for the brain?: the neuroprotective activities of the female sex hormone' (Google eBook), Springer, 2001, p2

29. http://www.drlam.com/articles/estrogen_dominance.asp

30. Vliet Elizabeth Lee, 'It's My Ovaries, Stupid!', Simon and Schuster, 2003, p249

31. http://www.ehow.com/about_4577601_symptoms-estrogen-dominance.html

32. Kohlstadt Ingrid, 'Scientific Evidence for Musculoskeletal, Bariatric, and Sports Nutrition', (Google eBook), CRC Press, 2006, p243

33. http://www.ehow.com/about_4577601_symptoms-estrogen-dominance.html

34. http://www.estrogendominanceguide.com/saliva-testing-for-estrogen-dominance

35. http://www.virginiahopkinstestkits.com/interpretsaliva.html

36. http://www.virginiahopkinstestkits.com/hormonebloodspot.html

37. Hall, DC, 'Nutritional influences on oestrogen metabolism', Applied Nutritional Science Reports, 200, 2001, p1-p8

38. Jackson Nisha, Rouzier Neal, 'The Hormone Survival Guide for Perimenopause: Balance Your Hormones Naturally', Larkfield Publishing, 2004, p22

39. Hudson Tori, Northrup Christiane, 'Women's Encyclopaedia of Natural Medicine: Alternative Therapies and Integrative Medicine', McGraw-Hill Professional, 1999, p164

40. Hudson Tori, Northrup Christiane, 'Women's Encyclopaedia of Natural Medicine: Alternative Therapies and Integrative Medicine', McGraw-Hill Professional, 1999, p164

41. http://www.ehow.com/facts_5091008_natural-supplements-boost-progesterone.html

42. Rao, 'Textbook of Gynaecology', Elsevier, India, 2008, p134

43. Henriette A, Delemarre-Van de Waal, 'Abnormalities in Puberty: Scientific and Clinical Advances', Karger Publishers, 2005, p143

44. Daftary & Patki, 'Reproductive Endocrinology & Infertility', BI Publications, 2009, p192

45. Balen AH, Conway GS, Kaltsas G, et al, 'Polycystic ovary syndrome: the spectrum of the disorder in 1741 patients', Human Reproduction, 10, 1995, p2107-p2111.

46. Gangar Elizabeth, 'Gynecological Nursing: A Practical guide', Elsevier Health Sciences, 2001, p67

47. Dunne Nancy, Slater William, 'The Natural Diet Solution for PCOS and Infertility: How to Manage Poly Cystic Ovary Syndrome Naturally', Natural Solutions for PCOS, 2006, p68

48. http://www.gfmer.ch/Endo/Lectures_08/sexual_hormones.htm

49. Coelingh Bennink HJT, Vemer HM, 'Chronic Hyperandrogenic Anovulation', Taylor & Francis, 1990, p29

50. Diamanti-Kandarakis Evanthia, Nestler John E, 'Insulin Resistance and Poly Cystic Ovarian Syndrome: Pathogenesis, Evaluation, and Treatment', (Google eBook), Humana Press, 2007, p245

51. Carlson Karen J, Eisenstat Stephanie A, Ziporyn Terra Diane, 'The New Harvard Guide to Women's Health', Harvard University Press, 2004, p288

52. http://www.labtestsonline.org/understanding/analytes/prolactin/test.html

53. http://www.vitamins-supplements.org/hormones/DHEA.php

54. Zawadski J, Dunaif A, 'Diagnostic criteria for polycystic ovary syndrome: towards a rational approach', In: Dunaif A, Given J, Haseltine F, Merriam G, eds, Polycystic Ovary Syndrome. Cambridge, MA, Blackwell Scientific Publications, 1992, p377

55. DeVane GW, Czekala NM, Judd HL, Yen SS, 'Circulating gonadotropins, estrogens, and androgens in polycystic ovarian disease', American Journal of Obstetrics and Gynecology, 1975, 121 p496

56. White, Donna, 'The Hormone Makeover', Xulon Press, 2010, p152

57. Janssen OE, Mehlmauer N, Hahn S, Offner AH, Gartner R, 'High Prevalence of Autoimmune Thyroiditis in Patients with Polycystic Ovary Syndrome', European Journal of Endocrinology, Vol 150, Issue 3, 2004, p363-p369

58. Iervasi Giorgio, Pingitore Alessandro, 'Thyroid and Heart Failure: From Pathophysiology to Clinics', (Google eBook), Springer, 2009, p153

59. Krassas1 GE, Pontikides N, Kaltsas T, Papadopoulou P, 'Disturbances of menstruation in hypothyroidism', Clinical Endocrinology, Vol 50, Issue 5, May 1999, p655–p659

60. Wu P, Winter, 'Thyroid Disease and Diabetes', Clinical Diabetes. Vol 18, No 1, 2000, p38-p42

61. McQade C, Skugor M, Brennan DM, Hoar B, Stevenson C, Hoogwerf BJ, 'Hypothyroidism and Moderate Subclinical Hypothyroidism Are Associated with Increased All-Cause Mortality Independent of Coronary Heart Disease Risk Factors: A Precis Database Study', Thyroid, (8), July 2011, p837-p843

62. Stampfer MJ, Malinow MR, Wilert WC, Newcomer LM, Upson B, Ullmann D, 'A Prospective Study of Plasma Homocyst(e)ine and Risk of Myocardial Infarction in US Physicians', JAMA, 268(7), 1992, p877-p881

63. Stampfer MJ, Malinow MR, Wilert WC, Newcomer LM, Upson B, Ullmann D, 'A Prospective Study of Plasma Homocyst(e)ine and Risk of Myocardial Infarction in US Physicians', JAMA, 268(7), 1992, p877-p881

64. Ting RZ, Szeto CC, Chan MH, Ma KK, Chow KM, 'Risk Factors of Vitamin B12 Deficiency in Patients Receiving Metformin', Arch Intern Med, 166, 2006, p1975-p1979

65. Wile DJ, Toth C, 'Association of Metformin, Elevated Homocysteine, and Methylmalonic Acid Levels and Clinically Worsened Diabetic Peripheral Neuropathy', Diabetes Care, Vol 33 No 1, January 2010, p156-p161

66. Desouza C, Keebler M, McNamara DB, Fonseca V, 'Drugs Affecting Homocysteine Metabolism: Impact on Cardiovascular Risk', Drugs, Vol 62, No 4, 1, April 2002, p605-p616(12)

67. Atamer A, Demir B, Bayhan G, Atamer Y, Ilhan N, Akkus Z, 'Serum Levels of Leptin and Homocysteine in Women with Poly Cystic Ovary Syndrome and its Relationship to Endocrine, Clinical and Metabolic Parameters', The Journal of International Medical Research, Vol 36, No 1, Jan-Feb 2008, p96-p105

68. Dr Dingle, November 2009 Newsletter

69. Fonarow GC, Horwich TJ, 'Cholesterol and Mortality in Heart Failure: the Bad Gone Good?', Journal of the American College of Cardiology, 42, 2003, p1941-p1943

70. Ulmer H, Kelleher C, Diem G, Concin H, 'Why Eve is Not Adam: Prospective Follow up in 149,650 Women and Men of Cholesterol and Other Risk Factors Related to Cardiovascular and All-cause Mortality', Journal of Women's Health (Larchmt), 13(1), January-February 2004, p41-p53

CHAPTER 4 REFERENCES

1. Bagchi Debasis, 'Nutraceutical and Functional Food Regulations in the United States and Around the World', (Google eBook), Academic Press, 2008, p19

2. Preedy Victor, Watson Ronald Ross, Patel Vinood, 'Flour and Breads and Their Fortification in Health and Disease Prevention', (Google eBook), Academic Press, 2011, p264

3. Kovács Gábor T, Norman Robert, 'Dietary Approaches and Alternative Therapies for Poly Cystic Ovary Syndrome', Poly Cystic Ovary Syndrome, Cambridge University Press, 2007, p263

4. Goldman Marlene B, Hatch Maureen, 'Women and Health', Gulf Professional Publishing, 2000, pP279

5. Mittal Satish, 'The Metabolic Syndrome in Clinical Practice', (Google eBook), Springer, 2007, p56

6. Kotsirilos Vicki, Vitetta Luis, Sali Avni, 'A Guide to Evidence-Based Integrative and Complementary Medicine', Elsevier Australia, 2011, p530

7. Murray Frank, Saputo Len, 'Natural Supplements for Diabetes: Practical and Proven Health Suggestions for Types 1 and 2 Diabetes', Basic Health Publications, Inc, 2007, p113

8. Anton SD, et al, 'Effects of Chromium Picolinate on Food Intake and Satiety', Diabetes Technology & Therapeutics, 10(5), October 2008, p405-p412

9. Anderson et al. 'Elevated intakes of supplemental Chromium improve glucose and insulin variables in individuals with type 2 Diabetes', Diabetes, 46(11), Nov 1997, p1786-p1791

10. Dodson David, Mitchell Deborah R, 'The Diet Pill Guide: The Consumer's Book of Over-the-Counter and Prescription Weight-Loss Pills and Supplements', Macmillan, 2001, p57

11. Keane Maureen, Chace Daniella, Lung John A, 'What to Eat If You Have Diabetes: Healing Foods that Help Control Your Blood Sugar', McGraw-Hill Professional, 2006, p156

12. 'Healing with Vitamins', Hinkler Holistic Healing, Hinkler Books, 2005, Australia, p12

13. Pathak P, Kapoor SK, Kapil U, Dwivedi SN, 'Serum Magnesium Level Amongst Pregnant Women In A Rural Community of Haryana State, India', European Journal of Clinical Nutrition 2003, 57, p1504–p1506

14. Lopez-Ridaura Ruy, Willett Walter C, Rimm Eric B, Liu Simin, Stampfer Meir J, Manson JoAnn E, Hu Frank B, 'Magnesium Intake and Risk of Type 2 Diabetes in Men and Women', Diabetes Care, Vol 27, No 1, January 2004, p34-p140

15. Murray Frank, Saputo Len, 'Natural Supplements for Diabetes: Practical and Proven Health Suggestions for Types 1 and 2 Diabetes', Basic Health Publications, Inc, 2007, p117

16. Song Yiqing et al, 'Magnesium Intake, C-Reactive Protein, and the Prevalence of Metabolic Syndrome in Middle-Aged and Older U.S. Women', Diabetes Care, Vol 28, No 6, June 2005, p1438-p1444

17. Muneyyirci-Delale O, Nacharaju VL, Dalloul M, Jalou S, Rahman M, Altura BM, Altura BT, 'Divalent cations in women with PCOS: implications for cardiovascular disease', Gynecol Endocrinol, 15(3), 2002, p198-p201

18. Young Robert O, Young Shelley Redford, 'The PH Miracle for Diabetes: The Revolutionary Diet Plan for Type 1 and Type 2 Diabetics', (Google eBook), Hachette Digital Inc, 2004

19. Kotsirilos Vicki, Vitetta Luis, Sali Avni, 'A Guide to Evidence-Based Integrative and Complementary Medicine', Elsevier Australia, 2011, p521

20. Challem Jack, 'User's Guide to Nutritional Supplements', (Google eBook), Basic Health Publications, 2003, p10

21. Young Robert O, Young Shelley Redford, 'The PH Miracle for Diabetes: The Revolutionary Diet Plan for Type 1 and Type 2 Diabetics', (Google eBook), Hachette Digital Inc, 2004

22. Jones Marjorie Hurt, 'The Allergy Self-help Cookbook: Over 350 Natural Food Recipes, Free of all Common Food Allergens', Rodale, 2001, p55

23. Chimienti Fabrice, Favier Alain, Seve Michel, 'ZnT-8, A Pancreatic Beta-Cell-Specific Zinc Transporter', BioMetals, Vol 18, No 4, August 2005, p313-p317

24. Prasad Ananda S, 'Clinical, immunological, anti-inflammatory and antioxidant roles of zinc?', Experimental Gerontology, Vol 43, Issue 5, May 2008, p370-p377

25. Harris Colette, Cheung Theresa, 'PCOS and Your Fertility', (Google eBook), by Hay House, Inc, 2004, p40

26. Merson Michael H, Black Robert E, Mills Anne, 'International Public Health: Diseases, Programs, Systems, and Policies', Jones & Bartlett Learning, 2006, p228

27. Murray Frank, Saputo Len, 'Natural Supplements for Diabetes: Practical and Proven Health Suggestions for Types 1 and 2 Diabetes', Basic Health Publications Inc, 2007, p129

28. Michaelsson Gerd, 'Serum zinc and retinol-binding protein in acne', British Journal of Dermatology, Vol 96, Issue 3, March 1977, p283–p286

29. Hemat R, 'Principles of orthomolecularism', Urotext, 2003, p33

30. Eby George A, 'Zinc treatment prevents dysmenorrhea', Medical Hypotheses, Vol 69, Issue 2, 2007, p297-p301

31. Hemat R, 'Principles of orthomolecularism', Urotext, 2003, p33

32. Kristy M, Walker W Allan, 'Zinc Deficiency in Inflammatory Bowel Disease', Nutrition, Vol 46, Issue 12, December 1988, p401-p408

33. Murray Frank, Saputo Len, 'Natural Supplements for Diabetes: Practical and Proven Health Suggestions for Types 1 and 2 Diabetes', Basic Health Publications Inc, 2007, p129

34. Pepea Salvatore, Marascoa Silvana F, Haasb Steven J, Sheeranb Freya L, Krumb Henry, Rosenfeld Franklin L, 'Coenzyme Q10 in cardiovascular disease', Mitochondrion, The Role of Coenzyme Q in Cellular Metabolism: Current Biological and Clinical Aspects, Vol 7, Supplement 1, June 2007, s154-s167

35. Dingle Associate Professor Peter, 'Putting Statins In Perspective', ACNEM Journal, Vol 28, Dec 2009

36. http://www.umm.edu/altmed/articles/omega-6-000317.htm

37. Calder Philip C, 'n–3 Polyunsaturated fatty acids, inflammation, and inflammatory diseases', American Journal of Clinical Nutrition, Vol 83, No 6, June 2006, s1505-s1519

38. Spiller Gene A, 'Handbook of lipids in human nutrition', CRC Press, 1996, p68

39. Lake James, 'Textbook of Integrative Mental Health Care', Thieme, 2006

40. Popp-Snijders C, Schouten JA, Heine RJ, van der Meer J, van der Veen EA, 'Dietary supplementation of omega-3 polyunsaturated fatty acids improves insulin sensitivity in non-insulin-dependent diabetes', Diabetes Res.4(3), March 1987, p141-p147

41. Preedy Victor R, Watson Ronald Ross, Patel Vinood B, 'Nuts and seeds in health and disease prevention', (Google eBook), Academic Press, 2011, p151

42. Saldeen Pia, Saldeen Tom, 'Women and Omega-3 Fatty Acids', Obstetrical & Gynaecological Survey, Vol 59, Issue 10, October 2004, p722-p730

43. Long Cheryl, Keiley Lynn, 'Is Agribusiness Making Food Less Nutritious?', Mother Earth News, Ogden Publications, June-July 2004

44. http://www.guardian.co.uk/lifeandstyle/2005/may/15/foodanddrink.shopping3

45. http://www.organicconsumers.org/articles/article_18006.cfm

46. http://www.time.com/time/health/article/0,8599,1880145,00.html

47. Holford Patrick, 'The New Optimum Nutrition Bible', Random House Digital Inc, 2005, p32

48. Long Cheryl, Keiley Lynn, 'Is Agribusiness Making Food Less Nutritious?', Mother Earth News, Ogden Publications, June-July 2004

49. http://www.huffingtonpost.com/jeffrey-smith/genetically-modified-soy_b_544575.html

50. Healthy Child Healthy World, http://healthychild.org/live-healthy/checklist/limit_your_childs_intake_of_food_additives/

51. Challem Jack, 'Feed Your Genes Right: Eat to Turn Off Disease-causing Genes and Slow Down Aging', John Wiley & Sons, 2005, p14

52. Moran Lisa, Gibson-Helm Melanie, Teede Helena, Deeks Amanda, 'Polycystic ovary syndrome: a biopsychosocial understanding in young women to improve knowledge and treatment options', Journal of Psychosomatic Obstetrics & Gynecology, Vol 31, No 1, March 2010, p24-p31

CHAPTER 5 REFERENCES

1. Mathur R, Ko A, Hwang LJ, Low K, Azziz R, Pimentel M, 'Poly Cystic Ovary Syndrome is Associated with an Increased Prevalence of Irritable Bowel Syndrome', Digestive Diseases and Sciences, 55(4), April 2010, p1085-p1059

2. Kelly Chris CJ, Lyall Helen, Petrie John R, Gould Gwyn W, Connell John MC, Sattar Naveed, 'Low Grade Chronic Inflammation in Women with Poly Cystic Ovarian Syndrome', The Journal of Clinical Endocrinology & Metabolism, Vol 86, No 6, June 2001, p2453-p2455

3. Tarkun et al, 'Young Women with Polycystic Ovary Syndrome: Relationship with Insulin Resistance and Low-Grade Chronic Inflammation', The Journal of Clinical Endocrinology & Metabolism, Vol 89 No 11, November 2004, p5592-p5596

4. Zhang Xiaoqian, Essmann Michael, Burt Edward T, Larsen Bryan, 'Estrogen Effects on Candida Albicans: A Potential Virulence-Regulating Mechanism', The Journal of Infectious Diseases, 181, 2000, p1441-p1446

5. Berg Rodney D, 'Bacterial Translocation From the Gastrointestinal Tract', Trends in Microbiology, 3(4), April 1995, p149-p154

6. Naessen S, Carlstrom K, Garoff L, Glant R, Hirschberg A Linden, 'Poly Cystic Ovary Syndrome in Bulimic Women - an Evaluation Based on the New Diagnostic Criteria', Gynaecological Endocrinology, Vol 22, No 7, 2006, p388-p394

7. Ma1 Xiong, Hua1 Jing, Li Zhiping, 'Probiotics improve high fat diet-induced hepatic steatosis and insulin resistance by increasing hepatic NKT cells?', Journal of Hepatology, Volume 49, Issue 5, November 2008, p821-p830

8. Parnell JA, Reimer RA, 'Oligofructose, Prebiotic Weight loss during oligofructose supplementation is associated with decreased ghrelin and increased peptide YY in overweight and obese adults',Am J Clin Nutr, 89(6), 2009, p1751-p1759

9. Schiffrin Eduardo J, Parlesak Alexandr, Bode Christiane, Bode J Christian, van't Hof Martin A, Grathwohl Dominik, Guigoz Yves, 'Probiotic yogurt in the elderly with intestinal bacterial overgrowth: endotoxaemia and innate immune functions', British Journal of Nutrition, 2009, 101(7), p961-p966

10. Maslowski et al, 'Regulation of inflammatory responses by gut microbiota and chemoattractant receptor GPR43', Nature 461, 2009, p1282-p1286

11. DiBaise et al, 'Gut Microbiota and Its Possible Relationship With Obesity', Mayo Clinic Proceedings, Vol 83 No 4, April 2008, p460-p469

12. Daubioul et al, 'Dietary Fructans, but Not Cellulose, Decrease Triglyceride Accumulation in the Liver of Obese Zucker fa/fa Rats', The American Society for Nutritional Sciences J Nutr 132, 2002, p967-p973

13. Brzozowska MM, Ostapowicz G, Weltman MD, 'An Association Between Non-alcoholic Fatty Liver Disease and Poly Cystic Ovarian Syndrome', Journal of Gastroenterology & Hepatology, 24(2), Feb 2009, p243-p247

14. Cerda C, Pérez-Ayuso RM, Riquelme A, Soza A, Villaseca P, Sir-Petermann T, Espinoza M, Pizarro M, Solis N, Miquel JF, Arrese M, 'Non-alcoholic Fatty Liver Disease in Women with Poly Cystic Ovary Syndrome', Journal of Hepatology, Vol 47, Issue 3, September 2007, p412-p415

15. Daubioul et al, 'Dietary Fructans, but Not Cellulose, Decrease Triglyceride Accumulation in the Liver of Obese Zucker fa/fa Rats', The American Society for Nutritional Sciences J. Nutr. 132, 2002, p967-p973

16. Cani et al, 'Changes in gut microbiota control inflammation in obese mice through a mechanism involving GLP-2-driven improvement of gut permeability', Diabetes, 5(5), 2006, p1484-p1490

17. Gibson GR, Roberfroid MB, 'Dietary modulation of the human colonic microbiota: introducing the concept of prebiotics', J Nutr, 125(6), June 1995, p1401

18. Cani P et al, 'Metabolic endotoxemia initiates obesity and insulin resistance', Diabetes, 56, 2007, p1761-p1772

19. Muccioli Giulio G, Naslain Damien, Bäckhed Fredrik, Reigstad Christopher S, Lambert Didier M, Delzenne Nathalie M, Cani Patrice D, 'The endocannabinoid system links gut microbiota to adipogenesis', Molecular Systems Biology 6, Article No 392, July 2010

20. Neyrinck Audrey M, Possemiers Sam, Druart Céline, Van de Wiele Tom, De Backer Fabienne, Cani Patrice D, Larondelle Yvan, Delzenne Nathalie M, 'Prebiotic Effects of Wheat Arabinoxylan Related to the Increase in Bifidobacteria, Roseburia and Bacteroides/Prevotella in Diet-Induced Obese Mice', PLoS One, 6(6), 2011, e20944

21. Cani PD, Possemiers S, Van de Wiele T et al, 'Changes in gut microbiota control inflammation in obese mice through a mechanism involving GLP-2-driven improvement of gut permeability', Gut, 58, 2009, p1091–p1103

22. Cani Patrice D, Neyrinck Audrey M, Maton Nicole, Delzenne Nathalie M, 'Oligofructose Promotes Satiety in Rats Fed a High-Fat Diet: Involvement of Glucagon-Like Peptide-1', Obesity Research, 13, 2005, p1000-p1007

23. Wilders-Truschnig M, Mangge H, Lieners C, et al, 'IgG Antibodies Against Food Antigens are Correlated with Inflammation and Intima Media Thickness in Obese Juveniles', Exp Clin Endocrinol Diabetes, 116(4), April 2008, p241-p245

24. Backhed F, Manchester JK, Semenkovich CF, et al, 'Mechanisms Underlying the Resistance to Diet-induced Obesity in Germ-free Mice', Proceedings of the National Academy of Sciences USA, 104, 2007, p979-p984

25. Ley RE, Backhed F, Turnbaugh P, et al, 'Obesity Alters Gut Microbial Ecology', Proceedings of the National Academy of Sciences USA, 102, 2005, p11070-p11075

26. Backhed F, Ding H, Wang T, et al, 'The Gut Microbiota as an Environmental Factor that Regulates Fat Storage', Proceedings of the National Academy of Sciences USA, 101, 2004, p15718-p15723

27. Cani PD, Bibiloni R, Knauf C, et al, 'Changes in Gut Microbiota Control Metabolic Endotoxemia-induced Inflammation in High-fat Diet-induced Obesity and Diabetes in Mice', Diabetes, 57, 2008, p1470-p1481

28. Cani PD, Neyrinck AM, Fava F, et al, 'Selective Increases of Bifidobacteria in Gut Microflora Improve High-fat-diet-induced Diabetes in Mice Through a Mechanism Associated with Endotoxaemia', Diabetologia, 50, 2007, p2374-p2383

29. Cani PD, Knauf C, Iglesias MA, et al, 'Improvement of Glucose Tolerance and Hepatic Insulin Sensitivity by Oligofructose Requires a Functional Glucagon-like Peptide 1 Receptor', Diabetes, 55, 2006, p1484-p1490

30. Turnbaugh et al, 'A core gut microbiome in obese and lean twins', Nature, 457, Jan 2009, p480-p484

31. Sapone A, de Magistris L, Pietzak M, et al, 'Zonulin Upregulation is Associated with Increased Gut Permeability in Subjects with Type 1 Diabetes and Their Relatives', Diabetes, 55, 2006, p1443-p1449

CHAPTER 6 REFERENCES

1. Everly George S, Lating Jeffrey M, 'A Clinical Guide to the Treatment of the Human Stress Response', Springer, 2002, p51

2. Folkman Susan, Nathan Peter E, 'The Oxford Handbook of Stress, Health, and Coping', Oxford University Press US, 2010, p69

3. Kruger TF, Botha MH, 'Clinical Gynaecology', Juta and Company Ltd, 2008, p379

4. Carmina Enrico, Lobo Rogerio A, 'Polycystic Ovary Syndrome (PCOS): Arguably the Most Common Endocrinopathy Is Associated with Significant Morbidity in Women', The Journal of Clinical Endocrinology & Metabolism, Vol 84, No 6, 1999, p1897-p1899

5. Weiner L PhD, Primeau Margaret PhD, Ehrmann, David A MD, 'Androgens and Mood Dysfunction in Women: Comparison of Women With Polycystic Ovarian Syndrome to Healthy Controls', Psychosomatic Medicine 66, 2004, p356-p362

6. Diamanti-Kandarakis Evanthia, Economou Frangiskos, 'Stress in Women, Metabolic Syndrome and Polycystic Ovary Syndrome', Annals of the New York Academy of Sciences, Vol 1083, Stress, Obesity, and Metabolic Syndrome, November 2006, p54-p62

7. Interview with David Zava PhD, 'Cortisol Levels, Thyroid Function and Aging: How Cortisol Levels Affect Thyroid Function and Aging', Virginia Hopkins, Health Watch

8. Harris Colette, Cheung Theresa, 'The Ultimate PCOS Handbook: Lose Weight, Boost Fertility, Clear Skin and Restore Self-Esteem', Conari, 2008, p264

9. Shepherd Richard, Raats Monique, 'The Psychology of Food Choice', Volume 3, CABI, 2006, p124

10. Carmina Enrico, LoboRogerio A, 'Use of fasting blood to assess the prevalence of insulin resistance in women with polycystic ovary syndrome', Fertility and Sterility, Vol 82, Issue 3, September 2004, p661-p665

11. Speroff Leon, FritzMarc A, 'Clinical Gynaecologic Endocrinology and Infertility', Lippincott Williams & Wilkins, 2005, p479

12. Hannon Ruth A, Pooler Charlotte, Porth Carol Mattson, 'Porth Pathophysiology: Concepts of Altered Health States', Lippincott Williams & Wilkins, 2009, p495

13. Kumar Sudhesh, 'Obesity and Diabetes', John Wiley & Sons, 2009, p252

14. Levine T Barry, Levine Arlene B, 'Metabolic Syndrome and Cardiovascular Disease', Elsevier Health Sciences, 2006, p122

15. Hemat RAS, 'Orthomolecularism: Principles And Practice', Urotext, 2004, p540

16. Kraw Maia, 'Diagnosing Hyperandrogenism in Women', Endocrinology Rounds, Vol 6, Issue 2, February 2006

17. Talbott Shawn, 'The Cortisol Connection: Why Stress Makes You Fat and Ruins Your Health – And What You Can Do About It', Hunter House, 2007, p70

18. Tsatsoulis Agathocles, Wyckoff Jennifer Ann, Brown Florence M, 'Diabetes in Women: Pathophysiology and Therapy', Springer Japan Co Ltd, 2009, p182

19. Azziz Ricardo, Nestler John E, Dewailly Didier, 'Androgen Excess Disorders in Women: Poly Cystic Ovary Syndrome and Other Disorders', Humana Press, 2006, p355

20. McCook Judy Griffin, Reame Nancy E, Thatcher Samuel S, 'Health-Related Quality of Life Issues in Women With Polycystic Ovary Syndrome', Journal of Obstetric, Gynecologic, & Neonatal Nursing, Vol 34, Issue 1, January 2005, p12-p20

21. http://commons.pacificu.edu/cgi/viewcontent.cgi?article=1258&context=spp

22. Hyman Mark A MD, Editorial, 'The Life Cycles Of Women: Restoring Balance', Altern Ther Health Med, 13(3), 2007, p10-p16

23. Jin Putai, 'Efficacy of Tai Chi, brisk walking, meditation, and reading in reducing mental and emotional stress', Journal of Psychosomatic Research, Vol 36, Issue 4, May 1992, p361-p370

24. Ryu Hoon et al, 'Acute Effect of Qigong Training on Stress Hormonal Levels in Man', The American Journal of Chinese Medicine (AJCM), Vol 24, Issue 2, 1996, p193-p198

25. Stener-Victorin Elisabet, et al, 'Effects of Electro-Acupuncture on Nerve Growth Factor and Ovarian Morphology in Rats with Experimentally Induced Polycystic Ovaries', Biology of Reproduction, Vol 63 No 5, November 1 2000, p1497-p1503

26. Stener-Victorin Elisabet, et al, 'Acupuncture in Polycystic Ovary Syndrome: Current Experimental and Clinical Evidence', Journal of Neuroendocrinology, Volume 20, Issue 3, March 2008, p290-p298

27. www.yourspine.com/Chiropractic/Chiropractic%20Improves%20Brain%20Fbunction.aspx

28. Herzog W, Scheele D, Conway PJ, 'Electromyographic Responses of Back and Limb Muscles Associated with Spinal Manipulative Therapy', Spine, Jan 15; 24(2), p146-p152

29. http://www.altmd.com/Articles/Chiropractic-Care-for-Stress

30. Craggs-Hinton Christine, Balen Adam, 'Positive Options for Poly Cystic Ovary Syndrome: Self-help and Treatment', Hunter House, 2004, p85

31. Kenta Kimura, 'l-Theanine reduces psychological and physiological stress responses', Biological Psychology, Vol 74, Issue 1, January 2007, p39-p45

32. Lamothe Denise, 'The Taming of the Chew: A Holistic Guide to Stopping Compulsive Eating', (Google eBook), Penguin, 2002

CHAPTER 7 REFERENCES

1. Nitsche K, Ehrmann DA, 'Obstructive sleep apnea and metabolic dysfunction in polycystic ovary syndrome', Best Pract Res Clin Endocrinol Metab, 24(5), Oct 2010, p717-p730

2. Koopman RJ; Swofford SJ; Beard MN; Meadows SE, 'Obesity and metabolic disease', Prim Care, 36(2), June 2009, p257-p270

3. Miranda PJ; DeFronzo RA; Califf RM; Guyton JR, 'Metabolic syndrome: definition, pathophysiology, and mechanisms', Am Heart J, 149(1), Jan 2005, p33-p45

4. Harrison DG; Gongora MC, 'Oxidative stress and hypertension', Med Clin North Am, 93(3), May 2009, p621-p635

5. Pashkow FJ, Watumull DG, Campbell CL, 'Astaxanthin: a novel potential treatment for oxidative stress and inflammation in cardiovascular disease', Am J Cardiol, 101(10A), May 2008, 58D-68D

6. Tsimikas S, 'In vivo markers of oxidative stress and therapeutic interventions', Am J Cardiol, 101(10A), May 2008, 34D-42D

7. Ritchie RH, 'Evidence for a causal role of oxidative stress in the myocardial complications of insulin resistance', Heart Lung Circ, 18(1), Feb 2009, p11-p18

8. Libby P, Plutzky J, 'Inflammation in diabetes mellitus: role of peroxisome proliferator-activated receptor-alpha and peroxisome proliferator-activated receptor-gamma agonists', Am J Cardiol, 99(4A), Feb 2007, 27B-40B

9. Rajasingam D, Seed PT, Briley AL, Shennan AH, Poston L, 'A prospective study of pregnancy outcome and biomarkers of oxidative stress in nulliparous obese women', Am J Obstet Gynecol 200(4), 395, April 2009, e1-9

10. Gallagher EJ, LeRoith D, Karnieli E, 'The metabolic syndrome from insulin resistance to obesity and diabetes', Endocrinol Metab Clin North Am; 37(3), Sep 2008, p559-p579, vii

11. Agarwal A, Sharma RK, Desai NR, Prabakaran S, Tavares A, Sabanegh E, 'Role of oxidative stress in pathogenesis of varicocele and infertility', Urology, 73(3), March 2009, p461-p469

12. Kennedy S, Bergqvist A, Chapron C, et al, 'ESHRE guideline for the diagnosis and treatment of endometriosis', Hum Reprod 20, (10), 2005, p2698-p2704

13. Saito H, Seino T, Kaneko T, Nakahara K, Toxa M, Kurachi H, 'Endometriosis and oocyte quality'. Gynecol Obstet Invest, 53 (Suppl), 2002, p46-p51

14. Shelton RC, Miller AH, 'Eating ourselves to death (and despair): the contribution of adiposity and inflammation to depression', Prog Neurobiol, 91(4), August 2010, p275-p99

15. Dawood T, Schlaich MP, 'Mediators of target organ damage in hypertension: focus on obesity associated factors and inflammation', Minerva Cardioangiol, 57(6), Dec 2009, p687-p704b

16. Kolb H, Mandrup-Poulsen T, 'The global diabetes epidemic as a consequence of lifestyle-induced low-grade inflammation', Diabetologia, 53(1), Jan 2010, p10-p20

17. Devasagayam TP, Tilak JC, Boloor KK, Sane KS, Ghaskadbi SS, Lele RD, 'Free radicals and antioxidants in human health: current status and future prospects', J Assoc Physicians India, 01, 52, Oct 2004, p794-p804

18. Bayir H, 'Reactive oxygen species', Crit Care Med, 33 (12 Suppl), Dec 2005, s498-50

19. Reid MB, Jan 2008, 'Free radicals and muscle fatigue: Of ROS, canaries, and the IOC', Free Radic Biol Med, 44(2), Jan 2008, p169-p179

20. Ai Pham-Huy Lien, He Hua, Pham-Huyc Chuong, 'Free Radicals, Antioxidants in Disease and Health', International Journal of Biomedical Science 4(2), Jun 15 2008, p89-p96

21. Droge W, 'Free Radicals in the Physiological Control of Cell Function', Physiol Rev Vol 82, No 1, January 2002, p47-p95

22. Fedarko NS, 'The biology of aging and frailty', Clin Geriatr Med, 27(1), Feb 2011, p27-p37

23. Godbout JP, Johnson RW, 'Age and neuroinflammation: a lifetime of psychoneuroimmune consequences', Immunol Allergy Clin North Am, 29(2), May 2009, p321-p337

24. Ronzio RA, Pizzorno JE, Murray MT, (eds), 'Naturally Occurring Antioxidants', Textbook of Natural Medicine, Chapter 109, 2006

25. Menditatta S, Qu ZC, May JM, 'Erythrocyte ascorbate recycling: antioxidant effects in blood', Free Radic Biol Med, 15, 24(5), March 1998, p789-p797

26. May JM, Qu ZC, Whitesell RR, 'Ascorbic acid recycling enhances the antioxidant reserve of human erythrocytes', Biochemistry, 3, 34(39), Oct 1995, p12721-p12728

27. Dunne J, Caron A, Menu P, Alayash AI, Buehler PW, Wilson MT, Silaghi-Dumitrescu, R, Faivre B, Cooper, CE, 'Ascorbate removes key precursors to oxidative damage by cell-free haemoglobin in vitro and in vivo', Biochem J, 1, 399(3), Nov 2006, p513-p524

28. Frei B, England L, Ames BN, 'Ascorbate is an outstanding antioxidant in human blood plasma', Proc Natl Acad Sci USA, 86, 1989, p6377-p6381

29. Chan AC, 'Partners in defense, vitamin E and vitamin C', Can J Physiol Pharmacol, 71, 1993, p725-p731

30. Bruno RS, Leonard SW, Atkinson J, et al, 'Faster plasma vitamin E disappearance in smokers is normalized by vitamin C supplementation', Free Radic Biol Med, 40(4), 2006, p689-p697

31. Chan TY, 'Food-borne nitrates and nitrites as a cause of methemoglobinemia', Southeast Asian J Trop Med Public Health, 27, 1996, p189-p192

32. Rangan C, Barceloux DG, 'Food additives and sensitivities', Dis Mon, 55(5), May 2009, p292-p311

33. Ho SM, 'Environmental epigenetics of asthma: an update', J Allergy Clin Immunol, 126(3), Sep 2010, p453-p465

34. Smith Jr SC, Clark LT, Cooper RS, et al, 'Discovering the full spectrum of cardiovascular disease: Minority Health Summit 2003: report of the Obesity, Metabolic Syndrome, and Hypertension Writing Group', Circulation 111, (10), 2005, e134-e139

35. Koopman RJ, Swofford SJ, Beard MN, Meadows SE, 'Obesity and metabolic disease', Prim Care, 36(2), June 2009, p257-p270

36. Mehra R, Redline S, 'Sleep apnea: a proinflammatory disorder that coaggregates with obesity', J Allergy Clin Immunol, 121(5), May 2008, p1096-p1102

37. Horton R, 'The neglected epidemic of chronic disease', Lancet, 366, (9496), 2005, p1514

38. Strong, Mathers C, Leeder S, Beaglehole R, 'Preventing Chronic Diseases: How Many Lives Can We Save' Lancet, 2005, 366, 2005, p1578-p1582

39. Murray S, 'Doubling the burden: chronic disease', CMAJ, 174(6), March 2006, p771

40. Drewnowski A, Popkin BM, 'The nutrition transition: new trends in the Global Diet', Nutr Rev 55 (2), 1997, p31-p43

41. Popkin BM, Nielsen SJ, 'The sweetening of the world's diet', Obesity Res 11 (11), 2003, p1325-p1332

42. http://www.reuters.com/article/2009/01/06/us-usa-chronicidUSTRE5050S920090106?sp=true

43. Olshansky SJ, et al, 'Potential decline in life expectancy in the United States in the 21st century', N Engl J Med, 352(11), March 2005, p1138-p1145

44. Schauss AG, 'Fish Oils (Omega-3 Fatty Acids, Docosahexanoic Acid, Eicosapentaenoic Acid, Dietary Fish, and Fish Oils)' Chapter 94, from Pizzorno, Textbook of Natural Medicine, 3rd ed, 2006

45. Simopoulos AP, 'Evolutionary aspects of diet, the Omega-6/Omega-3 ratio and genetic variation: nutritional implications for chronic diseases', Biomed Pharmacother, 60(9), Nov 2006, p502-p507

46. Harris W, 'Omega-6 and Omega-3 fatty acids: partners in prevention', Curr Opin Clin Nutr Metab Care, 13(2), Mar 2010, p125-p129

47. Simopoulos AP, 'The importance of the Omega-6/Omega-3 fatty acid ratio in cardiovascular disease and other chronic diseases', ExpBiol Med (Maywood) 233(6), June 2008, p674-p688

48. O'Keefe JH Jr, Cordain L, 'Cardiovascular disease resulting from a diet and lifestyle at odds with our Paleolithic genome: how to become a 21st-century hunter-gatherer', Mayo Clin Proc, 2004 (1), Jan 79, p101-p108

49. Simopoulos AP, 'The importance of the ratio of omega-6/omega-3 essential fatty acids', Biomedicine & Pharmacotherapy, Vol 56, Issue 8, October 2002, p365-p379

50. O'Keefe JH Jr, Cordain L, 'Cardiovascular disease resulting from a diet and lifestyle at odds with our Paleolithic genome: how to become a 21st-century hunter-gatherer', Mayo Clin Proc, 2004 (1), Jan 79, p101-p108

CHAPTER 8 REFERENCES

1. Wilson D, 'Fear in the Fields', The Seattle Times, July 3, 4 and 13 (1997), collective reprint

2. Agency for Toxic Substances and Disease Registry (http://www.atsdr.cdc.gov/toxprofiles/tp46-c1-b.pdf)

3. Goldman L, Shannon M, 'Mercury in the Environment: Implications for Pediatricians', American Academy of Pediatrics Technical Report, Pediatrics, 108, 2001, p197-p205

4. Eil C, Nisula BS, 'The Binding Properties of Pyrethroids to Human Skin Fibroblast Androgen Receptors and to Sex Hormone Binding Blobulin', Journal of Steroid Biochemistry, 35, 1990, p409-p414

5. http://www.cancerschmancer.org/articles/environment/study-finds-toxic-chemicals-pregnant-womens-bodies

6. Fernandez SV, Russo J, 'Estrogen and Xenoestrogens in Breast Cancer', Toxicology & Pathology, Vol 38, No 1, January 2010, p110-p122

7. Déchaud H, et al, 'Xenoestrogen Interaction with Human Sex Hormone-Binding Globulin (hSHBG)', Steroids, PubMed, 64(5), May 1999, p328-p334

8. Lemasters GK, et al, Workshop to Identify Critical Windows of Exposure for Children's Health: Reproductive Health in Children and Adolescents Work Group Summary, Environmental Health Perspectives, 108 (Suppl 3), 2000, p505-p509

9. 'Women with Poly Cystic Ovary Syndrome Have Higher BPA Blood Levels, Study Finds', The Endocrine Society, Science Daily, 25 June 2010

CHAPTER 9 REFERENCES

1. 'Thyroid Disease: Understanding Hypothyroidism and Hyperthyroidism', Harvard Medical School, Health Publications Group, Harvard Health Publications, 2010, p7

2. Choksi Neepa Y, Jahnke Gloria D, St. Hilaire Cathy, Shelby Michael, 'Role of Thyroid Hormones in Human and Laboratory Animal Reproductive Health', Birth Defects Research (Part B) 68, 2003, p479-p491

3. Janssen OE, Mehlmauer N, Hahn S, Offner AH, Gartner R, 'High Prevalence of Autoimmune Thyroiditis in Patients with Poly Cystic Ovary Syndrome', European Journal of Endocrinology, Vol 150, Issue 3, 2004, p363-p369

4. Ghosh Subhadra, Kabir Syed N, Pakrashi Anita, Chatterjee Siddhartha, Chakravarty Baidyanath, 'Subclinical Hypothyroidism: A Determinant of Poly Cystic Ovary Syndrome', Research In Paediatrics, Horm Res, 39, 1993, p61-p66

5. Diamanti-Kandarakis Evanthia, Nestler John E, 'Insulin Resistance and Poly Cystic Ovarian Syndrome: Pathogenesis, Evaluation, and Treatment', Humana Press, 2007, p325

6. Lazarus John, Pirags Valdis, Butz Sigrid, 'The Thyroid and Reproduction', Georg Thieme Verlag, 2009, p74

7. Rosenthal M Sara, 'The Thyroid Sourcebook', McGraw-Hill Professional, 2008, p53

8. Warren Heymann, 'Thyroid Disorders with Cutaneous Manifestations', Springer, 2008, p11

9. Despopoulos Agamemnon, Silbernagl Stefan, 'Colour Atlas of Physiology', Pt 471, Thieme, 2000, p288

10. 'Fundamentals Physiology - A Textbook for Nursing Students', Jaypee Brothers Publishers, p222

11. De Pergola G, Ciampolillo A, Paolotti S, Trerotoli P, Giorgino R, 'Free triiodothyronine and thyroid stimulating hormone are directly associated with waist circumference, independently of insulin resistance, metabolic parameters and blood pressure in overweight and obese women', Clinical Endocrinology, Volume 67, Issue 2, August 2007, p265-p269

12. 'Fundamentals Physiology - A Textbook for Nursing Students', Jaypee Brothers Publishers, p224

13. Heymann Warren, 'Thyroid Disorders with Cutaneous Manifestations', Springer, 2008, p126-p127

14. Carr Bruce R, Blackwell Richard E, Azziz Ricardo, 'Essential Reproductive Medicine', McGraw-Hill Professional, 2005, p340

15. Williams Sue Rodwell, Schlenker Eleanor D, 'Essentials of Nutrition and Diet Therapy', Vol 1, Elsevier Health Sciences, 2003, p179

16. Despopoulos Agamemnon, Silbernagl Stefan, 'Colour Atlas of Physiology', Pt 471, Thieme, 2003, p288

17. Fritz Marc A, Speroff Leon, 'Clinical Gynaecologic Endocrinology and Infertility', Lippincott Williams & Wilkins, 2010, p893

18. Ghosh Subhadra, Kabir Syed N, Pakrashi Anita, Chatterjee Siddhartha, Chakravarty Baidyanath, 'Subclinical Hypothyroidism: A Determinant of Poly Cystic Ovary Syndrome', Research In Paediatrics, Horm Res, 39, 1993, p61-p66

19. Janssen OE, Mehlmauer N, Hahn S, Offner AH, Gartner R, 'High Prevalence of Autoimmune Thyroiditis in Patients with Poly Cystic Ovary Syndrome', European Journal of Endocrinology, Vol 150, Issue 3, 2004, p363-p369

20. Wartofsky Leonard, Dickey Richard A, 'The Evidence for a Narrower Thyrotropin Reference Range Is Compelling', The Journal of Clinical Endocrinology & Metabolism, Vol 90 No 9, September 2005, p5483-p5488

21. Walsh John P, Bremner Alexandra P, Feddema Peter, Leedman Peter J, Brown Suzanne J, O'Leary Peter, 'Thyrotropin and Thyroid Antibodies as Predictors of Hypothyroidism: A 13-Year, Longitudinal Study of a Community-Based Cohort Using Current Immunoassay Techniques', The Journal of Clinical Endocrinology & Metabolism, Vol 95, No 3, March 2010, p1095-p1104

22. Falcone Tommaso, Hurd William W, 'Clinical Reproductive Medicine and Surgery', Elsevier Health Sciences, 2007, p325

23. Nyström Ernst, Berg Gertrud EB, Jansson Svante KG, Torring Ove, Valdemarsson Stig V, 'Thyroid Disease in Adults', Springer, 2010, p127

24. 'Thyroid Dysfunction in Pregnancy: Optimising Foetal and Maternal Outcomes', Expert Review of Endocrinology & Metabolism, 5.4, July 2010, (9) p521

25. Fritz Marc A, Speroff Leon, 'Clinical Gynaecologic Endocrinology and Infertility', Lippincott Williams & Wilkins, 2010, p1, p214

26. Casey Brian M MD, Dashe Jodi S MD, Wells C Edward MD, McIntire Donald D PhD, Byrd William PhD, Leveno Kenneth J MD, Cunningham F Gary MD, 'Subclinical Hypothyroidism and Pregnancy Outcomes', Obstetrics & Gynecology, Vol 105, Issue 2, February 2005, p239-p224

27. Valentino Rossella, et al, 'Prevalence of Celiac Disease in Patients with Thyroid Autoimmunity,' Hormone research in pediatrics, Vol 51, No 3, 1999, p124-p127

28. Metcalfe Dean D, Sampson Hugh A, Simon Ronald A, 'Food Allergy: Adverse Reactions to Food and Food Additives', Wiley-Blackwell, 2003, p321

29. Abramson Jeremy, Stagnaro-Green Alex, 'Thyroid Antibodies and Foetal Loss: An Evolving Story', Thyroid, 11(1), January 2001, p57-p63

30. http://www.wilsonssyndrome.com

31. Cabot S, Jasinska M, 'Your Thyroid Problems Solved', Hero Productions, 2006

32. 'Case Studies for Complementary Therapists', Elsevier Australia, p148

33. Eales JG, 'The influence of nutritional state on thyroid function in various vertebrates', Integrative and Comparative Biology, Vol 28, Issue 2, 1988, p351-p362

34. FAQs About Iodine Nutrition, The Australian Thyroid Foundation (2008), http://www.thyroidfoundation.com.au/events/event_taw/taw_iodine.html. Date accessed 27.11.10

35. Boyages S, 'Clinical review 49: iodine deficiency disorders', J Clin Endocrinol Metab, 77, 1993, p587-p591

36. Eastman CJ, 'Iodine supplementation: the benefits for pregnant and lactating women in Australia and New Zealand', O & G (RANZCOG), 7(1 Autumn), 2005, p65-p66

37. de Benoist B, McLean E, Andersson M, Rogers L, 'Iodine deficiency in 2007: global progress since 2003', Food Nutr Bull, 29(3), 2008, p195-p202

38. http://baumannutrition.com/pdfs/thyroid.pdf

CHAPTER 10 REFERENCES

1. Sloan RP, Bagiella E, Powell T, 'Spirituality and Medicine', Religion, The Lancet, 353, (9153), 1999, p664-p667

2. Jarrett LS, 'Nourishing Destiny: The Inner Tradition of Chinese Medicine', Spirit Path Press, Stockbridge Massachusetts, 2001, p204-p208

3. Pert CB, 'Type 1 and Type 2 Opiate Receptor Distribution in Brain - What Does it Tell Us?', Advances in Biochemical Psychopharmacology, 28, 1981, p117-p131

4. Domar AD, Clapp D, 'Impact of Group Psychological Interventions on Pregnancy Rates in Infertile Women', Fertility and Sterility, 74 (1), July 2000, p190

5. http://www.time.com/time/health/article/0,8599,1951968,00.html

6. Gerstein MB, Bruce C, Rozowsky JS, Zheng D, Du J, Korbel JO, Emanuelsson O, Zhang ZD, Weissman S, Snyder M, 'What is a Gene, Post-ENCODE?', History and updated definition, Genome Research 17, 2007, p669-p681

7. Vercelli D, 'Epigenetics, and the Environment: Switching, Buffering, Releasing', Journal of Allergy and Clinical Immunology, 113(3), March 2004, p381

8. Verma M, Srivastava S, 'Epigenetics in Cancer: Implications for Early Detection and Prevention', The Lancet Oncology 3(12), 2002, p755-p763

9. Clark RSB, Bayir H, Jenkins LW, 'Posttranslational Protein Modifications', Critical Care Medicine, 33(12 Suppl), Dec 2005, s407-s409

10. Stover PJ, Caudill MA, 'Genetic and Epigenetic Contributions to Human Nutrition and Health: Managing Genome-diet Interaction', Journal of the American Dietetic Association, 108(9), September 2008, p1480-p1487

11. Afman L, Müller M, 'Nutritional Genomics: From Molecular Nutrition to Prevention of Disease', Journal of the American Dietetic Association, 106, 2006, p569-p576

12. Barnes S, 'Nutritional Genomics, Polyphenols, Diets, and Their Impact on Dietetics', Journal of the American Dietetic Association, 108(11), November 2008, p1888-p1895

13. Stover PJ, 'Physiology of Folate and Vitamin B12 in Health and Disease', Annual Review of Nutrition 62, (6 Pt 2), 2004, s3-s12

14. De Marco P, Moroni A, Merello E, de Franchis R, Andreussi L, Finnell RH, Barber RC, Cama A, Capra V, 'Folate Pathway Gene Alterations in Patients With Neural Tube Defects', American Journal of Medical Genetics, 95, 2000, p216-p223

15. Newnham JP, Pennell CE, Lye SJ, Rampono J, Challis JR, 'Early Life Origins of Obesity', Obstetrics & Gynaecology Clinics of North America, 36(2), June 2009, p227-p244, xii

16. Crocker MK, Yanovski JA, 'Pediatric obesity: etiology and treatment', Endocrinology Metabolism Clinics of North America, 38(3), September 2009, p525-p548

17. Simmons RA, 'Developmental Origins of Adult Disease', Pediatric Clinics of North America, 56(3), June 2009, p449-p466

18. Bagot RC, Meaney MJ, 'Epigenetics and the Biological Basis of Gene X Environment Interactions', Journal of American Academy of Child and Adolescent Psychiatry, 49(8), August 2010, p752-p771

19. Wright RJ, 'Epidemiology of Stress and Asthma: From Constricting Communities and Fragile Families to Epigenetics', Immunology Allergy Clinics of North America, 31(1), February 2011, p19-p39

20. Gicquel C, El-Osta A, Le Bouc Y, 'Epigenetic Regulation and Foetal Programming', Best Practice & Research: Clinical Endocrinology & Metabolism, 22(1), February 2008, p1-p16

21. Ogren MP, Lombroso PJ, 'Epigenetics: Behavioural Influences on Gene Function, Part I - Maternal Behaviour Permanently Affects Adult Behaviour in Offspring', Journal of American Academy of Child & Adolescent Psychiatry, 47(3), March 2008, p240-p244

22. Ogren MP, Lombroso PJ, 'Epigenetics: Behavioural Influences on Gene Function, Part II - Molecular Mechanisms', Journal of American Academy of Child & Adolescent Psychiatry, 47(4), April 2008, p374-p378

23. Ornish D, et al, 'Increased Telomerase Activity and Comprehensive Lifestyle Changes: a Pilot Study', Lancet Oncology, 9(11), November 2008, p1048-p1057

24. Ornish D, Magbanua MJ, Weidner G, Weinberg V, Kemp C, Green C, Mattie MD, Marlin R, Simko J, Shinohara K, Haqq CM, Carroll PR, 'Changes in Prostate Gene Expression in Men Undergoing an Intensive Nutrition and Lifestyle Intervention', Proceedings of the National Academy of Sciences US, 105(24), June 2008, p8369-p8374

25. Frattaroli J, Weidner G, Dnistrian AM, Kemp C, Daubenmier JJ, Marlin RO, Crutchfield L, Yglecias L, Carroll PR, Ornish D, 'Clinical Events in Prostate Cancer Lifestyle Trial: Results From Two Years of Follow up', Urology, 72(6), December 2008, p1319-p1323

26. Liepa GU, Sengupta A, Karsies D, 'Poly Cystic Ovary Syndrome (PCOS) and Other Androgen Excess-related Conditions: Can Changes in Dietary Intake Make a Difference?', Nutrition in Clinical Practice, 23(1), February 2008, p63-p71

27. Tomlinson J, Millward A, Stenhouse E, Pinkney J, 'Type 2 Diabetes and Cardiovascular Disease in Poly Cystic Ovary Syndrome: What are the Risks and Can They Be Reduced?', Diabetic Medicine, 27(5), May 2010, p498-p515

28. Moran LJ, Noakes M, Clifton PM, Norman RJ, 'The Effect of Modifying Dietary Protein and Carbohydrate in Weight Loss on Arterial Compliance and Postprandial Lipidemia in Overweight Women with Poly Cystic Ovary Syndrome', Fertility and Sterility, 94(6), November 2010, p2451-p2454

29. Lipton B, 'The Biology of Belief', Mountain of Love Books, US, 2005

30. Lipton B, Bhaerman S, 'Spontaneous Evolution: Our Positive Future (and a Way to Get There From Here)', Hay House, US, 2009

31. Church Dawson, 'The Genie in Your Genes: Epigenetic Medicine and the New Biology of Intention', (Google eBook), Elite Books, 2009

32. http://uhs.berkeley.edu/lookforthesigns/depressionsuicide.shtml

33. Harvey BH, 'Is Major Depressive Disorder a Metabolic Encephalopathy?', Human Psychopharmacology, 23(5), July 2008, p371-p384

34. Malhi GS, Parker GB, Greenwood J, 'Structural and Functional Models of Depression: From Sub-types to Substrates', Acta Psyciatrica Scandinavica, 111(2), February 2005, p94-p105

35. Bondy B, 'Pharmacogenomics in Depression and Antidepressants', Dialogues in Clinical Neuroscience, 7(3), January 2005, p223-p230

36. Scheffer RE, 'Psychopharmacology: Clinical Implications of Brain Neurochemistry', Pediatric Clinics of North America, 53(4), August 2006, p767-p775

37. Hu Y, Russek SJ, 'BDNF and the Diseased Nervous System: a Delicate Balance Between Adaptive and Pathological Processes of Gene Regulation', Journal of Neurochemistry, 105(1), April 2008, p1-p17

38. aan het Rot M, Mathew SJ, Charney DS, 'Neurobiological Mechanisms in Major Depressive Disorder', Canadian Medical Association Journal, 180(3), February 2009, p305-p313

39. Mischoulon D, 'Update and Critique of Natural Remedies as Antidepressant Treatments', Psychiatric Clinics of North America, 30(1), 1 March 2007, p51-p68

40. Adams SM, Miller KE, Zylstra RG, 'Pharmacologic Management of Adult Depression, American Family Physician', 77(6), March 2008, p785-p792

41. Shyn SI, Hamilton SP, 'The Genetics of Major Depression: Moving Beyond the Monoamine Hypothesis', Psychiatric Clinics of North America, 33(1), March 2010, p125-p140

42. http://www.mayoclinic.com/health/depression/MH00035

43. Deechera D, et al, 'From Menarche to Menopause: Exploring the Underlying Biology of Depression in Women Experiencing Hormonal Changes', Psychoneuroendocrinology, 33:3 2008

44. Wilkins KM, Warnock JK, Serrano E, 'Depressive Symptoms Related to Infertility and Infertility Treatments', Psychiatric Clinics of North America, 33(2), June 2010, p309-p321

45. Rasgon NL, Rao RC, Hwang S, Altshuler LL, Elman S, Zuckerbrow-Miller J, Korenman SG, 'Depression in Women with Poly Cystic Ovary Syndrome: Clinical and Biochemical Correlates', Journal of Affective Disorders, 74(3), May 2003, p299-p304

46. Deeks AA, Gibson-Helm ME, Teede HJ, 'Anxiety and Depression in Poly Cystic Ovary Syndrome: a Comprehensive Investigation', Fertility and Sterility, 93(7), May 2010, p2421-p2423

47. Hollinrake E, Abreau A, Maifield M, et al, 'Increased Risk of Depressive Disorders in Women with Poly Cystic Ovary Syndrome', Fertility and Sterility, 87, 2007, p1369-p1376

48. Richardson MR, 'Current Perspectives in Poly Cystic Ovary Syndrome', American Family Physician, 68(4), August 2003, p697-p704

49. Kalro BN, Loucks TL, Berga SL, 'Neuromodulation in Poly Cystic Ovary Syndrome', Obstetric & Gynaecology Clinics of North America, 28(1), March 2001, p35-p62

50. http://www.medicinenet.com/anxiety/article.htm

51. http://www.nimh.nih.gov/health/topics/anxiety-disorders/index.shtml

52. Kirsch I, 'Challenging received wisdom: antidepressants and the placebo effect', McGill J Med 11(2), November 2008, p219-p222

CHAPTER 11 REFERENCES

1. Booth Frank W, Chakravarthy Manu V, Spangenburg Espen E, 'Exercise and gene expression: physiological regulation of the human genome through physical activity', J Physiol 1, 543 (Pt 2), September 2002, p399-p411

2. Eriksson J, Taimela S, Koivisto VA, 'Exercise and the metabolic syndrome', Diabetologia 40, 1997, p125-p135

3. Hamburg Naomi M, McMackin Craig J, Huang Alex L, Shenouda Sherene M, Widlansky Michael E, Schulz Eberhard, Gokce Noya, Ruderman Neil B, Keaney Jr John F, Vita Joseph A, 'Physical Inactivity Rapidly Induces Insulin Resistance and Microvascular Dysfunction in Healthy Volunteers', Arteriosclerosis, Thrombosis, and Vascular Biology, 27, 2007, p2650-p2656

4. Randeva HS, Lewandowski KC, Drzewoski J, Brooke-Wavell K, O'Callaghan C, Czupryniak L, Hillhouse EW, Prelevic GM, 'Exercise Decreases Plasma Total Homocysteine in Overweight Young Women with Poly Cystic Ovary Syndrome', Journal of Clinical Endocrinology & Metabolism, 87, 2002, p4496

5. Dunaif A, 'Insulin Resistance and the Poly Cystic Ovary Syndrome: Mechanism and Implications for Pathogenesis', Endocrine Review, 18(6), 1997, p774-p800

6. 'Exercise Training Program May Be Helpful in Young Women with Poly Cystic Ovary Syndrome', Medscape Medical News, Journal of Clinical Endocrinology & Metabolism, 2007

7. Sabuncu T, Vural H, Harma M, 'Oxidative Stress in Poly Cystic Ovary Syndrome and its Contribution to the Risk of Cardiovascular Disease', Clinical Biochemistry, 34, 2001, p401-p413

8. Fenkci V, Fenkci S, Yilmazer M, Serteser M, 'Decreased Total Antioxidant Status and Increased Oxidative Stress in Women with Poly Cystic Ovary Syndrome May Contribute to the Risk of Cardiovascular Disease', Fertility and Sterility, 80, 2003, p123-p127

9. Hollinrake Elizabeth BS, Abreu Alison MD, Maifeld Michelle RNC, Van Voorhis Bradley J MD, Dokras Anuja MD, 'Increased Risk of Depressive Disorders in Women with Poly Cystic Ovary Syndrome', Fertility and Sterility, Vol 87, Issue 6, June 2007, p369-p376

10. Weiner Cindy L PhD, Primeau Margaret PhD, Ehrmann David A MD, 'Androgens and Mood Dysfunction in Women: Comparison of Women With Poly Cystic Ovarian Syndrome to Healthy Controls', Psychosomatic Medicine, 66, 2004, p356-p362

11. Vigorito C, et al, 'Beneficial Effects of a Three-month Structured Exercise Training Program on Cardiopulmonary Functional Capacity in Young Women with Poly Cystic Ovary Syndrome', Journal of Clinical Endocrinology & Metabolism, 92(4), 2007, p1379-p1384

12. Lee IM, Rexrode KM, Cook NR, Manson JE, Buring JE, 'Physical activity and coronary heart disease in women: is no pain, no gain passe?' JAMA 285, 2001, p1447-p1454

13. Huber-Buchholz MM, et al, 'Restoration of Reproductive Potential Lifestyle Modification in Obese Poly Cystic Ovary Syndrome: Role of Insulin Sensitivity and Luteinising Hormone', Journal of Clinical Endocrinology & Metabolism, 84(4), April 1999, p1470-p1474

14. Dr Trapp Gail, 'The Eight Second Secret', p15

15. Babraj John A, Vollaard Niels BJ, Keast Cameron, Guppy Fergus M, Cottrell Greg, Timmons James A, 'Extremely Short Duration High Intensity Interval Training Substantially Improves Insulin Action in Young Healthy Males', BMC Endocrine Disorders, 9:3 2009

16. Ibañez J, Izquierdo M, Argüelles I, Forga L, Larrión JL, García-Unciti M, Idoate F, Gorostiaga EM, 'Twice-weekly progressive resistance training decreases abdominal fat and improves insulin sensitivity in older men with type 2 diabetes', Diabetes Care; 28(3), March 2005, p662-p667

17. Kandel ER, Schwartz JH, Jessel TM, 'Principles of Neural Science', (4th edition), McGraw-Hill, 2000

18. Dr Chestnut James, 'Innate Physical Fitness & Hygiene', p81

19. Schutter Dennis JLG, Van Honk Jack, 'The Cerebellum on the Rise in Human Emotion', The Cerebellum, 4, 2005, p290-p294

20. Watson PJ, 'Non-motor Functions of the Cerebellum', Psychological Bulletin, Vol 85, No 5, 1978, p944-p967

21. http://www.yourspine.com/Chiropractic/Chiropractic%20Improves%20Brain%20Function.aspx

22. Char Sudhanva PhD, Carroll Lee PhD, 'Yoga as a Complement to Chiropractic Care', Journal of Vertebral Subluxation Research, July 2007, p1-p9

CHAPTER 12 REFERENCES

1. Falcone Tommaso, Hurd William W, 'Clinical Reproductive Medicine and Surgery', Elsevier Health Sciences, 2007, p283

2. Bolin Anne, Wheleha Patricia, 'Human sexuality: biological, psychological, and cultural perspectives', Taylor & Francis, 2009, p104

3. Tsatsoulis Agathocles, Wyckoff Jennifer Ann, Brown Florence M, 'Diabetes in Women: Pathophysiology and Therapy', Springer, 2009, p184

4. Farid Nadir R, Diamanti-Kandarakis Evanthia, 'Diagnosis and Management of Poly Cystic Ovary Syndrome ', (Google eBook), Springer, 2009, p182

5. Duggan Christopher, Watkins John B, Walker W. Allan, 'Nutrition in Pediatrics: Basic Science, Clinical Applications', PMPH-USA, 2008, p730

6. McCluskey S, Evans C, Lacey JH, Pearce JM, Jacobs H, 'Poly Cystic Ovary Syndrome and Bulimia', Fertility and Sterility, 55(2), 1991, p287-p291

7. Goldman Marlene B, Hatch Maureen, 'Women and Health', Gulf Professional Publishing, 2000, p208

8. Volek J, et al, 'Comparison of Energy-restricted Very Low carbohydrate and Low fat Diets on Weight Loss and Body Composition in Overweight Men and Women', Nutrition & Metabolism (London), 1(1):13, 2004

9. Dashti HM, et al, 'Beneficial Effects of a Ketogenic Diet in Obese Diabetic Subjects', Molecular & Cellular Biochemistry, 302(1-2), August 2007, p249-p256

10. Layman DK, et al, 'Dietary Protein and Exercise Have Additive Effects on Body Composition During Weight Loss in Adult Women', Nutrition, 135(8), 2005, p1903-p1910

11. Johnstone AM, Horgan GW, et al, 'Effects of a High-protein Ketogenic Diet on Hunger, Appetite, and Weight Loss in Obese Men Feeding Ad Libitum', American Journal of Clinical Nutrition, 87(1), 2008, p44-p55

12. Kasim-Karakas Sidika E, Almario Rogelio U, Cunningham Wendy, 'Effects of Protein Versus Simple Sugar Intake on Weight Loss in Poly Cystic Ovary Syndrome (According to the National Institutes of Health Criteria)', Fertility and Sterility, Vol 92, Issue 1, July 2009, p262-p270

13. Dunne Nancy, Slater William, 'The Natural Diet Solution for PCOS and Infertility: How to Manage Poly Cystic Ovary Syndrome Naturally', Natural Solutions for PCOS, 2006, p7

14. McDonald Lyle, 'The Ketogenic Diet: a Complete Guide for the Dieter and Practitioner', 1998, p67

15. Austin GL, Dalton CB, et al, 'A very low carbohydrate diet improves symptoms and quality of life in diarrhea-predominant irritable bowel syndrome', Clin Gastroenterol Hepatol, 7(6), June 2009, p706-p708

16. Austin GL, Dalton CB, et al, 'A very low carbohydrate diet improves symptoms and quality of life in diarrhea-predominant irritable bowel syndrome', Clin Gastroenterol Hepatol, 7(6), June 2009, p706-p708

17. Grodner Michele, Long Sara, DeYoung Sandra, 'Foundations and Clinical Applications of Nutrition: a Nursing Approach', Elsevier Health Sciences, 2004, p154

18. Halton Thomas L, Hu Frank B, 'The Effects of High Protein Diets on Thermogenesis, Satiety and Weight Loss: A Critical Review', J Am Coll Nutr, Vol 23, No 5, October 2004, p373-p385

19. Mozaffarian D, Katan MB, Ascherio A, Stampfer MJ, Willett WC, 'Trans Fatty Acids and Cardiovascular Disease', New England Journal of Medicine, 354 (15), 2006, p1601-p1613

20. Hu FB, van Dam RM, Liu S, 'Diet and Risk of Type II Diabetes: the Role of Types of Fat and Carbohydrate', Diabetologia, 44 (7), 2001, p805-p817

21. Kavanagh K, Jones KL, Sawyer J, Kelley K, Carr JJ, Wagner JD, Rudel LL, 'Trans Fat Diet Induces Abdominal Obesity and Changes in Insulin Sensitivity in Monkeys', Obesity, Silver Spring, 15 (7), July 2007, p1675-p1684

22. Chavarro Jorge E, Rich-Edwards Janet W, Rosner Bernard A, Willett Walter C, 'Dietary Fatty Acid Intakes and the Risk of Ovulatory Infertility', American Journal of Clinical Nutrition, 85 (1), January 2007, p231-p237

23. Roan Shari, 'Trans Fats and Saturated Fats Could Contribute to Depression', Sydney Morning Herald, 28 January 2011

24. Blundell JE, Findlayson G, 'Is susceptibility to weight gain characterised by homeostatic or hedonic risk factors for overconsumption?', Physiol Behav 82, 2004, p21-p25

25. http://www.whfoods.com/genpage.php?tname=nutrient&dbid=84

26. Frassetto LA, Morris RC, Sebastian A, 'A practical approach to the balance between acid production and renal excretion in humans', J Nephrol, 19 (suppl 9), 2006, p533-p540

27. Carroll Angela, 'Optimal Protocols for Weight Control', The 2010 Metagenics International Congress, Melbourne, p41

28. Kirchengast S, Huber J, 'Body Composition Characteristics and Body Fat Distribution in Lean Women with Poly Cystic Ovary Syndrome', Human Reproduction, 16 (6), 2001, p1255-p1260

29. Good Candace, Tulchinsky Mark, Mauger David, Demers Laurence M, Legro Richard S, 'Bone Mineral Density and Body Composition in Lean Women with Poly Cystic Ovary Syndrome', Fertility and Sterility, Vol 72, Issue 1, July 1999, p21-p25

30. Nestler John E, Jakubowicz Daniela J, 'Lean Women with Poly Cystic Ovary Syndrome Respond to Insulin Reduction with Decreases in Ovarian P450c17a Activity and Serum Androgens', The Journal of Clinical Endocrinology & Metabolism, Vol 82, No 12, December 1997, p4075-p4079

31. Covington Sharon N, Burns Linda Hammer, 'Infertility counselling: a comprehensive handbook for clinicians', Cambridge University Press, 2006, p189

32. Strauss Jerome F, Barbieri Robert L, 'Yen and Jaffe's reproductive endocrinology: physiology, pathophysiology, and clinical management', Elsevier Health Sciences, 2009, p522

33. Zellner D, Loaiza S, Gonzalez Z, Pita J, Morales J, Pecora D, Wolf A, 'Food Selection Change Under Stress, Physiology & Behaviour', Vol 87, Issue 4, April 2006, p789-p793

34. Oliver G, Wardle J, 'Perceived Effects of Stress on Food Choice', Physiology & Behaviour, Vol 66, Issue 3, May 1999, p511-p515

35. Moberg E, Kollind M, Lins PE, Adamson U, 'Acute Mental Stress Impairs Insulin Sensitivity in IDDM Patients, Diabetologia', Vol 37, No 3, 1994, p247-p251

CHAPTER 13 REFERENCES

1. Tsatsoulis Agathocles, Wyckoff Jennifer Ann, Brown Florence M, 'Diabetes in Women: Pathophysiology and Therapy', (Google eBook), Springer, 2009, p142

2. Editorial by Balen Adam H, Dresner Martin, 'Should Obese Women with Poly Cystic Ovary Syndrome Receive Treatment for Infertility?', British Medical Journal, 23 February 2006; 332: 434 doi: 10.1136/bmj.332.7539.434.

3. Leppert Phyllis Carolyn, Peipert Jeffrey F, 'Primary Care for Women', Lippincott Williams & Wilkins, 2003, p250

4. Carrell Douglas T, 'Reproductive Endocrinology and Infertility: Integrating Modern Clinical and Laboratory Practice', (Google eBook), Springer, 2010, p149

5. Garg, 'Mastering the Presbyopic Surgery Lenses & Phakic IOLS', Jaypee Brothers Publishers, p255

6. Tsatsoulis Agathocles, Wyckoff Jennifer Ann, Brown Florence M, 'Diabetes in Women: Pathophysiology and Therapy', (Google eBook), Springer, 2009, p182

7. http://chattychiro.com/?page_id=10

8. Diamanti-Kandarakis Evanthia, Nestler John E, 'Insulin Resistance and Poly Cystic Ovarian Syndrome: Pathogenesis, Evaluation, and Treatment', (Google eBook), Humana Press, 2007, p324

9. Diamanti-Kandarakis Evanthia, Nestler John E, 'Insulin Resistance and Poly Cystic Ovarian Syndrome: Pathogenesis, Evaluation, and Treatment', (Google eBook), Humana Press, 2007, p213–p215

10. Glover Timothy D, Barratt CLR, 'Male Fertility and Infertility', Cambridge University Press, 1999, p162

11. http://www.womenshealth.gov/faq/infertility.cfm#f

12. Desai Sadhna, Parihar Mandakini, Allahabadia Gautam, 'Infertility: Principles and Practice', BI Publications, 2003, p100

13. Laurent SL, Thompson SJ, Addy C, Garrison CZ, Moore EE, 'An epidemiologic study of smoking and primary infertility in women', Fertil Steril. 57(3), March 1992, p565-p572

14. Kesmodel Ulrik, Wisborg Kirsten, Olsen Sjúrdur Fródi, Henriksen Tine Brink, Secher Niels Jørgen, 'Moderate Alcohol Intake in Pregnancy and the Risk of Spontaneous Abortion', Alcohol and Alcoholism, 37 (1), 2002, p87-p92

15. Tikkanen Minna, Nuutila Mika, Hiilesmaa Vilho, Paavonen Jorma, Ylikorkala Olavi, 'Clinical Presentation and Risk Factors of Placental Abruption', Acta Obstetricia et Gynecologica Scandinavica, Vol 85, No 6, 2006, p700-p705

16. O'Leary Colleen M, Nassar Natasha, Zubrick Stephen R, Kurinczuk Jennifer J, Stanley Fiona, Bower Carol, 'Evidence of a Complex Association Between Dose, Pattern and Timing of Prenatal Alcohol Exposure and Child Behaviour Problems', Addiction, Vol 105, Issue 1, January 2010, p74-p86

17. Habermann Thomas M, 'Mayo Clinic Internal Medicine Concise Textbook', (Google eBook), Mayo Clinic, CRC Press, 2007, p883

18. Bryant Bronwen Jean, Knights Kathleen Mary, 'Pharmacology for Health Professionals', Elsevier Australia, 2010, p433

19. Mendelson JH, Mello NK, Ellingboe J, Skupny AS, Lex BW, Griffin M, 'Marijuana Smoking suppresses Luteinising Hormone in Women', Journal of Pharmacology and Experimental Therapeutics, Vol 237, No 3, June 1986, p862-p866

20. Smith DE, Moser C, Wesson DR, Apter M, Buxton ME, Davison JV, Orgel M, Buffum J, 'A Clinical Guide to the Diagnosis and Treatment of Heroin-related Sexual Dysfunction', Journal of Psychoactive Drugs, 14(1-2), January-June 1982, p91-p99

21. Thyer AC, King TS, Moreno AC, Eddy CA, Siler-Khodr TM, Schenken RS, 'Cocaine Impairs Ovarian Response to Exogenous Gonadotropins in Nonhuman Primates', Journal of the Society for Gynaecologic Investigation, 8(6), November-December 2001, p358- p362

22. Cwikela J, Gidronb Y, Sheinerc E, 'Psychological interactions with infertility among women', Vol 117, Issue 2, December 2004, p126-p131

23. Ciechanowska, Magdalena, 'Effect of Stress on the Expression of GnRH and GnRH Receptor (GnRH-R) Genes in the Preoptic Area-hypothalamus and GnRH-R Gene in the Stalk/Median Eminence and Anterior Pituitary Gland in Ewes During Follicular Phase of the Estrous Cycle', Acta Neurobiologiae Experimentalis, (0065-1400), 67 (1), January 2007, p1

24. Kelly Chris CJ, Lyall Helen, Petrie John R, Gould Gwyn W, Connell John MC, Sattar Naveed, 'Low Grade Chronic Inflammation in Women with Poly Cystic Ovarian Syndrome', The Journal of clinical endocrinology and metabolism, Vol 86, No 6, 2001, p2453-p2455

25. Vgontzasa Alexandros N, Trakadaa Georgia, Bixlera Edward O, Linb Hung-Mo, Pejovica Slobodanka, Zoumakisc Emmanuel, Chrousosc George P, Legro Richard S, 'Plasma Interleukin 6 Levels are Elevated in Poly Cystic Ovary Syndrome Independently of Obesity or Sleep Apnoea, Metabolism', Vol 55, Issue 8, August 2006, p1076-p1082

26. Gonzalez F, Thusu K, Abdel-Rahman E, Prabhala A, Tomani M, Dandona P, 'Elevated Serum Levels of Tumour Necrosis Factor Alpha in Normal-weight Women with Poly Cystic Ovary Syndrome', Metabolism, 48, 1999, p437-p441

27. Hotamisligil GS, Arner P, Caro JF, Atkinson RL, Spiegelman BM, 'Increased Adipose Tissue Expression of Tumour Necrosis Factor in Human Obesity and Insulin Resistance', Journal of Clinical Investigation, 95: 1995, p2409-p2415

28. Lee KS, et al, 'Relationships Between Concentrations of Tumour Necrosis Factor-alpha and Nitric Oxide in Follicular Fluid and Oocyte Quality', Journal of Assisted Reproduction and Genetics, 17, 2000, p222-p228

29. Krassas GE, Pontikides N, Kaltsas Th, Papadopoulou Ph, Paunkovic J, Paunkovic N, Duntas LH, 'Disturbances of Menstruation in Hypothyroidism', Clinical Endocrinology, 50, 1999, p655-p659

30. http://www.cumc.columbia.edu/dept/thyroid/pregnant.html

31. Zimmermann Michael MD, Burgerstein Lothar, 'Burgerstein's Handbook of Nutrition: Micronutrients in the Prevention and Therapy of Disease', Thieme, 2001, p231

32. Borchardt Kenneth A, Noble Michael A, 'Sexually Transmitted Diseases: Epidemiology, Pathology, Diagnosis, and Treatment', CRC Press, 1997, p42

33. Wilcox, Allen J, Dunson David, Baird Donna Day, 'The Timing of the Fertile Window in the Menstrual Cycle: Day Specific Estimates From A Prospective Study.' British Medical Journal. 321.7271, 2000

34. Parker Louise, 'Understanding and Treating PCOS', SGC Health, 2006, p8

35. http://medicalcentre.osu.edu/PatientEd/Materials/PDFDocs/women-in/preconception-care.pdf

36. Kopelman Peter G, Caterson Ian D, Dietz William H, 'Clinical Obesity in Adults and Children', (Google eBook), John Wiley and Sons, 2009, p241

37. Adamson Melitta Weiss, 'Food in Medieval Times', (Google eBook), Greenwood Publishing Group, 2004, p25

38. David Sami S, Blakeway Jill, 'Making Babies: A Proven 3-Month Program for Maximum Fertility', (Google eBook), Hachette Digital, 2009

39. Harris Colette, Cheung Theresa, 'PCOS and Your Fertility', (Google eBook), Hay House, 2004, p87

40. Northrup Christiane, 'Women's Bodies, Women's Wisdom: Creating Physical and Emotional Health and Healing', Random House, 2006, p424

41. Tamura H, Takasaki A, Miwa I, Taniguchi K, Maekawa R, Asada H, Taketani T, Matsuoka A, Yamagata Y, Shimamura K, Morioka H, Ishikawa H, Reiter RJ, Sugino N, 'Oxidative Stress Impairs Oocyte Quality and Melatonin Protects Oocytes From Free Radical Damage and Improves Fertilisation Rate', Journal of Pineal Research, 44(3), April 2008, p280-p287

42. Pillitteri Adele, 'Maternal & Child Health Nursing: Care of the Childbearing & Childrearing Family', Lippincott Williams & Wilkins, 2009, p315

43. Hipsley AH, 'Dietary Fibre and Pregnancy Toxaemia', British Medical Journal, Aug 22, 1953, p420

44. http://www.natural-progesterone-advisory-network.com/why-is-the-liver-so-important-in-hormone-balancing/

45. Evans Joel M, Aronson Robin, 'The Whole Pregnancy Handbook: an Obstetrician's Guide to Integrating Conventional and Alternative Medicine Before, During, and After Pregnancy', Penguin, 2005, p25

46. David Sami S, Blakeway Jill, 'Making Babies: A Proven 3-month Program for Maximum Fertility', (Google eBooks), Hachette Digital, 2009

47. Wilcox Allen J, 'Fertility and Pregnancy: an Epidemiologic Perspective', (Google eBook), Oxford University Press US, 2010, p28

48. Gangestad SW, Thornhill R, Garver CE, 'Changes in women's sexual interests and their partner's mate-retention tactics across the menstrual cycle: evidence for shifting conflicts of interest', Proc R Soc Lond B, Vol 269, No 1494, May 2002, p975-p982

49. Allen Wilcox J, 'The timing of the "fertile window" in the menstrual cycle: day specific estimates from a prospective study', BMJ, 321, 2000, p1259

50. Shaffer David R, Kipp Katherine, 'Developmental Psychology: Childhood and Adolescence', Cengage Learning, 2009, p139

CHAPTER 14 REFERENCES

1. Hantash B, et.al, Dermatologic Manifestations of Hirsutism, Medscape, http://emedicine.medscape.com/article/1072031-overview

2. Hudson, Tori ND, 'Women's Encyclopaedia of Natural Medicine', Keats Publishing, 1999, p142

3. Mishell Daniel Jr MD, 'Comprehensive Gynaecology', 3rd Ed, Mosby Publishing, 1997, p1087-p1099

4. Amoroso AM, ed, 'Unwanted Hair and Hirsutism: A Book for Women', Trafford Publishing, 2009, p71

5. Balen AH, 'Poly Cystic Ovary Syndrome: a Guide to Clinical Management', Taylor & Francis, 2005, p187

6. Chuan S, Chang J, 'Poly Cystic Ovary Syndrome and Acne', Skin Therapy Letter, 15(10), 2010, p1

7. Balen AH, 'Poly Cystic Ovary Syndrome: a Guide to Clinical Management', Taylor & Francis, 2005, p187

8. Teede H, et al, 'Poly Cystic Ovary Syndrome: a Complex Condition with Psychological, Reproductive and Metabolic Manifestations that Impacts on Health Across the Lifespan', BMC Medicine, 8, 2010, p41

9. Azziz R, et al, 'Androgen Excess Disorders in Women: Poly Cystic Ovary Syndrome and Other Disorders', Humana Press, 2006, p1714

10. Leppert PC, Peipert JF, 'Primary Care for Women', Lippincott Williams & Wilkins, 2003, p275

11. Velazquez EM, Mendoza S, Hamer T, Sosa F, Glueck CJ, 'Metformin therapy in polycystic ovary syndrome reduces hyperinsulinemia, insulin resistance, hyperandrogenemia, and systolic blood pressure, while facilitating normal menses and pregnancy', Metabolism, Vol 43, Issue 5, May 1994, p647-p654

12. http://www.nlm.nih.gov/medlineplus/ency/article/003148.htm

13. Homburg Roy, 'Should patients with polycystic ovarian syndrome be treated with metformin? A note of cautious optimism', Hum Reprod, 17 (4), 2002, p853-p856

14. Leung PCK, Adashi EY, 'The ovary', Academic Press, 2004, p502

15. Conn Jennifer J, Jacobs Howard S, 'Managing hirsutism in gynaecological practice', BJOG: An International Journal of Obstetrics & Gynaecology, Vol 105, Issue 7, July 1998, p687-p696

16. Smith Robyn N, Mann Neil J, Braue Anna, Mäkeläinen Henna, Varigos George A, 'A low-glycemic-load diet improves symptoms in acne vulgaris patients: a randomized controlled trial1,2,3', American Journal of Clinical Nutrition, Vol 86, No 1, July 2007, p107-p115

17. Hill P, Wynder E, 'Effect of a vegetarian diet and dexamethasone on plasma prolactin, testosterone and Dehydroepiandrosterone in men and women', Cancer Letters 7, 1979, p273-p282

18. Berrino Franco, Bellati Cristina, Secreto Giorgio, Camerini Edgarda, Pala Valeria, Panico Salvatore, Allegro Giovanni, Kaaks Rudolf, 'Reducing Bioavailable Sex Hormones Through a Comprehensive Change in Diet: the Diet and Androgens (DIANA) Randomised Trial', Cancer Epidemiol Biomarkers Prev, 10, January 2001, p25

19. Takahashi, Bergner P, 'Glycyrrhiza: Licorice root and testosterone', Medical Herbalism, 11(3), p11-p12

CHAPTER 15 REFERENCES

1. Setji TL, Brown AJ, 'Poly Cystic Ovary Syndrome: Diagnosis and Treatment', American Journal of Medicine, 120(2), February 2007, p128-p132

2. Azziz R, et al, 'The Androgen Excess and PCOS Society Criteria for the Poly Cystic Ovary Syndrome: the Complete Task Force Report', Fertility and Sterility, 91(2), February 2009, p456-p488

3. Giallauria F, Orio F, Palomba S, Lombardi G, Colao A, Vigorito C, 'Cardiovascular Risk in Women with Poly Cystic Ovary Syndrome', Journal of Cardiovascular Medicine (Hagerstown), 9(10), October 2008, p987-p992

4. Tomlinson J, Millward A, Stenhouse E, Pinkney J, 'Type 2 Diabetes and Cardiovascular Disease in Poly Cystic Ovary Syndrome: What are the Risks and Can They be Reduced?', Diabetic Medicine, 1, 27(5), May 2010, p498-p515

5. Diehl AM, 'Hepatic Complications of Obesity', Gastroenterology Clinics of North America, 39(1), March 2010, p57-p68

6. Atay V, Cam C, Muhcu M, Cam M, Karateke A, 'Comparison of Letrozole and Clomiphene Citrate in Women with Poly Cystic Ovaries Undergoing Ovarian Stimulation', Journal of International Medical Research, 34 (1), 2006, p73-p76

7. Dehbashi S, Vafaei H, Parsanezhad MD, Alborzi S, 'Time of Initiation of Clomiphene Citrate and Pregnancy Rate in Poly Cystic Ovarian Syndrome', International Journal of Gynaecology & Obstetrics, 93, (1), 2006, p44-p48

8. Palomba S, Orio Jr F, Falbo A, et al, 'Prospective Parallel Randomised, Double-blind, Double-dummy Controlled Clinical Trial Comparing Clomiphene Citrate and Metformin as the First-line Treatment for Ovulation Induction in Non-obese Anovulatory Women with Poly Cystic Ovary Syndrome', Journal of Clinical Endocrinology & Metabolism , 90, (7), 2005, p4068-p4074

9. Sahin Y, Yirmibes U, Kelestimur F, Aygen E, 'The Effects of Metformin on Insulin Resistance, Clomiphene-induced Ovulation and Pregnancy Rates in Women with Poly Cystic Ovary Syndrome', European Journal of Obstetrics & Gynaecology Reproduction Biology, 113, (2), 2004, p214-p220

10. Radosh L, 'Drug Treatments for Poly Cystic Ovary Syndrome', American Family Physician, 79(8), April 2009, p671-p676

11. Duranteau L, Lefevre P, Jeandidier N, Simon T, Christin-Maitre S, 'Should Physicians Prescribe Metformin to Women with Poly Cystic Ovary Syndrome PCOS?', Ann Endocrinol, (Paris), 71(1), February 2010, p25-p27

12. http://www.cdc.gov/ncbddd/features/Clomiphene-Citrate.html

13. http://www.rxlist.com/clomid-drug.htm#

14. Wulffele MG, Kooy A, Lehert P, Bets D, Ogterop JC, Borger Van Der Burg B, Donker AJ, Stehouwer CD, 'Effects of Short-term Treatment with Metformin on Serum Concentrations of Homocysteine, Folate and Vitamin B12 in Type 2 Diabetes Mellitus: a Randomised, Placebo-controlled Trial', Journal of Internal Medicine, 254(5), November 2003, p455-p463

15. http://naturaldatabase.therapeuticresearch.com

16. Pasquali R, Antenucci D, Casimirri F, et al, 'Clinical and Hormonal Characteristics of Obese Amenorrheic Hyperandrogenic Women Before and After Weight Loss', Journal of Clinical Endocrinology & Metabolism 68. (1), 1989, p173-p179

17. Bates G, Whitworth N, 'Effect of Body Weight Reduction on Plasma Androgens in Obese, Infertile Women', Fertility and Sterility, 38, (4), 1982, p406-p409

18. Moran L, Noakes M, Clifton P, 'Dietary Composition in Restoring Reproductive and Metabolic Physiology in Overweight Women with Poly Cystic Ovary Syndrome', Journal of Clinical Endocrinology & Metabolism, 88, 2003, p812-p819

19. Hamilton-Fairley D, Kiddy D, Anyaoku V, 'Response of Sex Hormone Binding Globulin and Insulin-like Growth Factor Binding Protein-1 to an Oral Glucose Tolerance Test in Obese Women with Poly Cystic Ovary Syndrome Before and After Calorie Restriction', Clinical Endocrinology (Oxf), 39, 1993, p363-p367

20. Kiddy D, Hamilton-Fairley D, Seppala M, 'Diet-induced Changes in Sex Hormone Binding Globulin and Free Testosterone in Women with Normal or Poly Cystic Ovaries: Correlation with Serum Insulin and Insulin-like Growth Factor-I', Clinical Endocrinology (Oxf), 31, 1989, p757-p763

21. Moran LJ, Hutchison SK, Norman RJ, Teede HJ, 'Lifestyle Changes in Women with Poly Cystic Ovary Syndrome, Cochrane Database Systematic Reviews', February 2011, 2:CD007506

22. Huber-Buchholz MM, Carey DGP, Norman RJ, 'Restoration of Reproductive Potential by Lifestyle Modification in Obese Poly Cystic Ovary Syndrome: Role of Insulin Sensitivity and Luteinising Hormone', Journal of Clinical Endocrinology & Metabolism, 84, 1999, p1470-p1474

23. Clark AM, Thornley B, Tomlinson L, et al, 'Weight Loss in Obese Infertile Women Results in Improvement in Reproductive Outcome for all Forms of Fertility Treatment', Human Reproduction, 13, 1998, p1502-p1505

24. Toscani MK, Mario FM, Radavelli-Bagatini S, Wiltgen D, Matos Cristina M, Spritzer Mara P, 'Effect of High-protein or Normal-protein Diet on Weight Loss, Body Composition, Hormone, and Metabolic Profile in Southern Brazilian Women with Poly Cystic Ovary Syndrome: a Randomised Study', Journal of Gynaecology Endocrinology, 27(11), May 2011, p925-p930

25. Farshchi H, Rane A, Love A, Kennedy RL, 'Diet and Nutrition in Poly Cystic Ovary Syndrome (PCOS): Pointers for Nutritional Management', Journal of Obstetrics & Gynaecology, 27(8), November 2007, p762-p773

26. Ornstein RM, Copperman NM, Jacobson MS, 'Effect of Weight Loss on Menstrual Function in Adolescents with Poly Cystic Ovary Syndrome', Journal of Pediatric and Adolescent Gynaecology, 24(3), June 2011, p161-p165

27. Dansinger ML, Gleason JA, Griffith JL, et al, 'Comparison of the Atkins, Ornish, Weight Watchers, and Zone diets for Weight Loss and Heart Disease Risk Reduction', Journal of the American Medical Association, 293, 2005, p43-p53

28. Marsh KA, Steinbeck KS, Atkinson FS, Petocz P, Brand-Miller JC, 'Effect of a Low Glycaemic Index Compared with a Conventional Healthy Diet on Poly Cystic Ovary Syndrome', American Journal of Clinical Nutrition, 92(1), July 2010, p83-p92

29. O'Keefe JH Jr, Cordain L, 'Cardiovascular Disease Resulting From a Diet and Lifestyle at Odds with our Paleolithic Genome: How to Become a 21st-century Hunter-gatherer', Mayo Clinic Proceedings, 79(1), January 2004, p101-p108

30. Simopoulos AP, 'Evolutionary Aspects of Diet, the Omega-6/Omega-3 Ratio and Genetic Variation: Nutritional Implications for Chronic Diseases', Biomedicine & Pharmacotherapy, 60(9), November 2006, p502-p507

31. Mathur R, Alexander CJ, Yano J, Trivax B, Azziz R, 'Use of Metformin in Poly Cystic Ovary Syndrome', American Journal of Obstetrics & Gynaecology, 199(6), December 2008, p596-p609

32. Salpeter SR, Buckley NS, Kahn JA, Salpeter EE, 'Meta-analysis: Metformin Treatment in Persons at Risk for Diabetes Mellitus', American Journal of Medicine, February 2008, 121(2), p149-p157, e2

33. Dwyer-Schull P, 'Nursing Spectrum Drug Handbook', McGraw Hill, 2008

34. Pfeifer SM, Kives S, 'Poly Cystic Ovary Syndrome in the Adolescent, Obstetric & Gynaecology', Clinics of North America, 36(1), March 2009, p129-p152

35. Rossi B, Sukalich S, Droz J, et al, 'Prevalence of Metabolic Syndrome and Related Characteristics in Obese Adolescents With and Without Poly Cystic Ovary Syndrome', Journal of Clinical Endocrinology & Metabolism, Vol 93, No 12, December 2008, p4780-p4786

36. Wild RA, Carmina E, Diamanti-Kandarakis E, Dokras A, Escobar-Morreale HF, Futterweit W, Lobo R, Norman RJ, Talbott E, Dumesic DA, 'Assessment of Cardiovascular Risk and Prevention of Cardiovascular Disease in Women with the Poly Cystic Ovary Syndrome: a Consensus Statement by the Androgen Excess and Poly Cystic Ovary Syndrome (AE-PCOS) Society', Journal of Clinical Endocrinology & Metabolism, 95(5), May 2010, p2038-p2049

37. Salley KE, Wickham EP, Cheang KI, Essah PA, Karjane NW, Nestler JE, 'Glucose Intolerance in Poly Cystic Ovary Syndrome - a Position Statement of the Androgen Excess Society', Journal of Clinical Endocrinology & Metabolism, 92(12), December 2007, p4546-p4556

38. Marsh K, Brand-Miller J, 'The Optimal Diet for Women with Poly Cystic Ovary Syndrome?', British Journal of Nutrition, 94(2), August 2005, p154-p165

39. Hu, Frank B, 'Overweight and Obesity in Women: Health Risks and Consequences', Journal of Women's Health, 12(2), February 2003, p163-p172

40. Visioli Francesco, Borsani Luisa, Galli Claudio, 'Diet and prevention of coronary heart disease: the potential role of phytochemicals', Cardiovasc Res, 47 (3), 2000, p419-p425

41. Solomon TPJ, Blannin AK, 'Effects of Short-term Cinnamon Ingestion on in Vivo Glucose Tolerance, Diabetes', Obesity and Metabolism 9, 2007, p895-p901

42. Mang B, Wolters M, Schmitt B, et al, 'Effects of a Cinnamon Extract on Plasma Glucose HbA, and Serum Lipids in Diabetes Mellitus Type 2', European Journal of Clinical Investigation 36, 2006, p340-p344

43. Khan A, Safdar M, Ali Khan MM, et al, 'Cinnamon Improves Glucose and Lipids of People with Type 2 Diabetes', Diabetes Care 26, (12), 2003, p3215-p3218

44. Najm W, Lie D, 'Herbals Used for Diabetes, Obesity, and Metabolic Syndrome', Primary Care, 37(2), June 2010, p237-p254

45. Leproult R, Copinschi G, Buxton O, et al, 'Sleep Loss Results in an Elevation of Cortisol Levels the Next Evening', Sleep 20, 1997, p865-p870

46. Spath-Schwalbe E, Gofferje M, Kern W, et al, 'Sleep Disruption Alters Nocturnal ACTH and Cortisol Secretory Patterns', Biological Psychiatry 29, 1991, p575-p584

47. Nitsche K, Ehrmann DA, 'Obstructive Sleep Apnoea and Metabolic Dysfunction in Poly Cystic Ovary Syndrome', Best Practice & Research: Clinical Endocrinology & Metabolism, 24(5), October 2010, p717-p730

48. Zhou XS, Rowley JA, Demirovic F, et al, 'Effect of Testosterone on the Apnoeic Threshold in Women During NREM Sleep', Journal of Applied Physiology 94, 2003, p101-p107

49. Regensteiner JG, Woodard WD, Hagerman DD, et al, 'Combined Effects of Female Hormones and Metabolic Rate on Ventilatory Drives in Women', Journal of Applied Physiology, 66, 1989, p808-p813

50. Schwab RJ, Pien GW, 'Sleep Disorders During Pregnancy', Sleep 27, 2004, p1405-p1417

51. Harsch IA, Schahin SP, Radespiel-Troger M, et al, 'Continuous Positive Airway Pressure Treatment Rapidly Improves Insulin Sensitivity in Patients with Obstructive Sleep Apnoea Syndrome', American Journal of Respiratory and Critical Care Medicine 169, 2004, p156-p162

52. Babu AR, Herdegen J, Fogelfeld L, et al, 'Type 2 Diabetes, Glycaemic Control, and Continuous Positive Airway Pressure in Obstructive Sleep Apnoea', Archives of Internal Medicine 165, 2005, p447-p452

53. Pizzorno JE, Murray MT, (eds), 'Menopause in Textbook of Natural Medicine', 3rd ed, Chapter 189, Elsevier, 2006

54. Schwartz ET, Holtorf K, 'Hormones in Wellness and Disease Prevention: Common Practices, Current State of the Evidence, and Questions for the Future', Primary Care, 35(4), December 2008, p669-p705

55. Grunstein RR, 'Metabolic Aspects of Sleep Apnoea', Sleep, 19(10 Suppl), December 1996, s218-s220

56. Nielsen LS, Danielsen KV, Sørensen TI, 'Short Sleep Duration as a Possible Cause of Obesity: Critical Analysis of the Epidemiological Evidence', Obesity Reviews, 12(2), February 2011, p78-p92

57. 'Weight Control and Physical Activity', IARC Handbooks of Cancer Prevention, The International Agency for Research on Cancer (WHO), IARC Press, 2002

58. Dossus L, Kaaks R, 'Nutrition, Metabolic Factors and Cancer Risk', Best Practice & Research: Clinical Endocrinology & Metabolism, 22(4), August 2008, p551-p571

59. Brinton LA, Moghissi KS, Westhoff CL, Lamb EJ, Scoccia B, 'Cancer Risk Among Infertile Women with Androgen Excess or Menstrual Disorders (Including Poly Cystic Ovary Syndrome)', Fertility and Sterility, 94(5), October 2010, p1787-p1792

60. Gammon M, Thompson W, 'Poly Cystic Ovaries and the Risk of Breast Cancer', American Journal of Epidemiology 134, 1991, p818-p824

61. Futterweit W, 'Poly Cystic Ovary Syndrome: a Common Reproductive and Metabolic Disorder Necessitating Early Recognition and Treatment', Primary Care, 34(4), December 2007, p761-p789, vi.

62. Unger J, ed, 'Diagnosing and Managing the Metabolic Syndrome in Adults, Children and Adolescents', Diabetes Management in Primary Care, Lippincott Williams and Wilkins, 2007, p43-p87

63. Kuhl H, 'Comparative Pharmacology of Newer Progestogens', Drugs, 51, 1996, p188-p215

64. Baillargeon JP, McClish DK, Essah PA, et al, 'Association Between the Current Use of Low Dose Oral Contraceptives and Cardiovascular Arterial Disease: a Meta-analysis', Journal of Clinical Endocrinology & Metabolism 90, (7), 2005, p3863-p3870

65. Sherif K, 'Benefits and Risks of Oral Contraceptives', American Journal of Obstetrics & Gynaecology, 180, (6 Pt 2), 1999, s343-s348

66. Basen-Engquist K, Chang M, 'Obesity and Cancer Risk: Recent Review and Evidence', Current Oncology Reports, 13(1), February 2011, p71-p76

67. Graves BW, 'The Obesity Epidemic: Scope of the Problem and Management Strategies', Journal of Midwifery & Women's Health, 55(6), November 2010, p568-p578

68. Hevener AL, Febbraio MA, 'Stock Conference Working Group, The 2009 Stock Conference Report: Inflammation, Obesity and Metabolic Disease', Obesity Reviews, 11(9), September 2010, p635-p644

69. Rana JS, Nieuwdorp M, Jukema JW, Kastelein JJ, 'Cardiovascular Metabolic Syndrome - an Interplay of, Obesity, Inflammation, Diabetes and Coronary Heart Disease', Diabetes, Obesity and Metabolism, 9(3), May 2007, p218-p232

70. Rosário Monteiro and Isabel Azevedo, 'Chronic Inflammation in Obesity and the Metabolic Syndrome,' Mediators of Inflammation,Volume 2010, p96-p105

71. Thaler JP, Schwartz MW, 'Minireview: Inflammation and Obesity Pathogenesis: the Hypothalamus Heats Up', Endocrinology, 151(9), September 2010, 4109-15 .

72. Nathan C, 'Epidemic Inflammation: Pondering Obesity', Molecular Medicine, 14(7-8), July 2008, p485-p492

73. Hollinrake E, Abreau A, Maifield M, et al, 'Increased Risk of Depressive Disorders in Women with Poly Cystic Ovary Syndrome', 87, 2007, p1369-p1376

74. Burns LH, 'Psychiatric Aspects of Infertility and Infertility Treatments', Psychiatric Clinics of North America, 30(4), December 2007, p689-p716

75. Loret de Mola JR, 'Obesity and its Relationship to Infertility in Men and Women', Obstetric & Gynaecology Clinics of North America, 36(2), June 2009, p333-p346

76. Deeks AA, Gibson-Helm AE, Teede HJ, 'Anxiety and Depression in Poly Cystic Ovary Syndrome: a Comprehensive Investigation', Fertility and Sterility, 93, (7), May 2010, p2421-p2423

77. Meller W, Burns LH, Crow S, et al, 'Major Depression in Unexplained Infertility', Journal of Psychosomatic Obstetric Gynaecology 23, 2002, p27-p30

78. Jones GL, Balen AH, Ledger WL, 'Health-related Quality of Life in PCOS and Related Infertility: How Can We Assess This?', Human Fertility, 11(3), September 2008, p173-p185

79. Jones GL, Hall JM, Balen AH, Ledger WL, 'Health-related Quality of Life Measurement in Women with Poly Cystic Ovary Syndrome: a Systematic Review', Human Reproduction Update, 14(1), January-February 2008, p15-p25

80. Janssen OE, Hahn S, Tan S, Benson S, Elsenbruch S, 'Mood and Sexual Function in Poly Cystic Ovary Syndrome', Seminars in Reproductive Medicine, 26(1), January 2008, p45-p52

81. Coffey S, Bano G, Mason HD, 'Health-related Quality of Life in Women with Poly Cystic Ovary Syndrome: a Comparison with the General Population Using the Poly Cystic Ovary Syndrome Questionnaire (PCOSQ) and the Short Form-36 (SF-36)', Journal of Gynaecology Endocrinology, 22(2), February 2006, p80-p86

82. Coffey S, Mason H, 'The Effect of Poly Cystic Ovary Syndrome on Health-related Quality of Life', Journal of Gynaecology Endocrinology, 17(5), October 2003, p379-p386

CHAPTER 17 REFERENCES

1. Winter, Joysa, 'Cinnamon Extract for Insulin Resistance', Functional Foods and Neutraceuticals, 2006, p42

2. Piatti PM, Monti F, Fermo I, Baruffaldi L, Nasser R, Santambrogio G, Librenti MC, Galli-Kienle M, Pontiroli AE, Pozza G, 'Hypocaloric high-protein diet improves glucose oxidation and spares lean body mass: comparison to hypocaloric high-carbohydrate diet', Metabolism, 43(12), 1994, p1481-p1487

3. Golay A, et al, 'Weight-Loss With Low or High Carbohydrate Diet?', International Journal of Obesity, 20 (12), 1996, p1067-p1072

4. Food and Drug Administration, http://www.mayoclinic.com/health/cholesterol/CL00002

CHAPTER 18 REFERENCES

1. Godsland IF, Walton C, Felton C, Proudler A, Patel A, Wynn V, 'Insulin Resistance, Secretion, and Metabolism in users of oral contraceptives', Journal of Clinical Endocrinology & Metabolism, Vol 74, p64-p70

2. Diamanti-Kandarakis E, Baillargeon P, Iuorno MJ, Jakubowicz D, Nestler JE, 'A Modern Medical Quandary: Polycystic Ovary Syndrome, Insulin Resistance, and Oral Contraceptive Pills', The Journal of Clinical Endocrinology & Metabolism, Vol 88, No 5, p1927-p1932

3. Ornish D, et al, 'Can lifestyle changes reverse coronary heart disease? The lifestyle heart trial', Lancet, July 21 1990, 336(8708), p129-p133

Made in the USA
Middletown, DE
16 January 2015